The Muhammad Ali
Parkinson Center
100 Questions &
Answers About
Parkinson Disease

Second Edition

Abraham Lieberman, MD
Muhammad Ali Parkinson Center
Phoenix, AZ

JONES AND BARTLETT PUBLISHERS
Sudbury, Massachusetts
BOSTON   TORONTO   LONDON   SINGAPORE

World Headquarters
Jones and Bartlett Publishers
40 Tall Pine Drive
Sudbury, MA 01776
978-443-5000
info@jbpub.com
www.jbpub.com

Jones and Bartlett Publishers
Canada
6339 Ormindale Way
Mississauga, Ontario L5V 1J2
Canada

Jones and Bartlett Publishers
International
Barb House, Barb Mews
London W6 7PA
United Kingdom

Jones and Bartlett's books and products are available through most bookstores and online booksellers. To contact Jones and Bartlett Publishers directly, call 800-832-0034, fax 978-443-8000, or visit our website at www.jbpub.com.

Substantial discounts on bulk quantities of Jones and Bartlett's publications are available to corporations, professional associations, and other qualified organizations. For details and specific discount information, contact the special sales department at Jones and Bartlett via the above contact information or send an email to specialsales@jbpub.com

The authors, editor, and publisher have made every effort to provide accurate information. However, they are not responsible for errors, omissions, or for any outcomes related to the use of the contents of this book and take no responsibility for the use of the products and procedures described. Treatments and side effects described in this book may not be applicable to all people; likewise, some people may require a dose or experience a side effect that is not described herein. Drugs and medical devices are discussed that may have limited availability controlled by the Food and Drug Administration (FDA) for use only in a research study or clinical trial. Research, clinical practice, and government regulations often change the accepted standard in this field. When consideration is being given to use of any drug in the clinical setting, the healthcare provider or reader is responsible for determining FDA status of the drug, reading the package insert, and reviewing prescribing information for the most up-to-date recommendations on dose, precautions, and contraindications, and determining the appropriate usage for the product. This is especially important in the case of drugs that are new or seldom used.

Production Credits
Executive Publisher: Christopher Davis
Editorial Assistant: Sara Cameron
Production Editor: Daniel Stone
V.P., Manufacturing and Inventory Control: Therese Connell
Manufacturing and Inventory Control Supervisor: Amy Bacus
Composition: Glyph International
Text Printing: Malloy, Inc.

Cover Credits
Cover Design: Carolyn Downer
Cover Printing: Malloy, Inc.
Cover Images: Top Photo: © forestpath/ShutterStock, Inc.; Bottom Left Photo: © Jostein Hauge/ShutterStock, Inc.; Bottom Right Photo: © Monkey Business Images/ShutterStock, Inc.

Library of Congress Cataloging-in-Publication Data
Lieberman, A. N. (Abraham N.), 1938-
    The Muhammad Ali Parkinson center 100 questions and answers
    about Parkinson disease/Abraham Lieberman.—2nd. ed.
        p. cm.
    Includes bibliographical references and index.
    ISBN-13: 978-0-7637-7253-6
    ISBN-10: 0-7637-7253-4
1. Parkinson's disease—Popular works. 2. Parkinson's disease—Miscellanea. I. Title. II. Title: 100 questions and answers about Parkinson disease.
    RC382.L543 2010
    616.8'33—dc22
                                        2009019555
6048

Printed in the United States of America
13 12 11 10   10 9 8 7 6 5 4 3 2

The second edition of *100 Questions & Answers About Parkinson Disease* is dedicated to Muhammad and Lonnie Ali, to Jimmy and Nancy Walker, and to Sean Curry and the staff of Celebrity Fight Night. Muhammad Ali needs no introduction. He's the most celebrated athlete of the century and the most recognizable person on earth. I have known Muhammad and Lonnie Ali for 20 years, since Muhammad was diagnosed with Parkinson disease. I have seen him battle the disease for 20 years, never giving in. It's "The Greatest's" greatest fight, greater than the "Thrilla in Manila" or the "Rumble in the Jungle." Muhammad's battle is summarized in a poem he and I wrote, which is reprinted in this book.

In 1998, Muhammad and Lonnie Ali joined with Jimmy Walker, a Phoenix philanthropist, to start Celebrity Fight Night. Each year, Celebrity Fight Night brings together athletes, businesspeople, entertainers, and good people from everywhere for a fundraiser to benefit the Muhammad Ali Parkinson Center (MAPC) at the Barrow Neurological Institute. "Fight Nighters" have included Kevin Costner, Billy Crystal, Michael J. Fox, Whitney Houston, Larry King, Barry Manilow, Phil Mickleson, Reba McIntire, Arnold Palmer, the Phoenix Suns, Arnold Schwarzenegger, Donald Trump, and Dionne Warwick. The money raised by these Celebrity Fight Nights have gone to the Muhammad Ali Parkinson Center to ensure that every patient who comes to the Center receives the same care that Muhammad Ali would receive. In these days of managed care, brief doctor visits, and little educational or emotional support for patients, MAPC is an oasis—a place where, because of Muhammad and Lonnie Ali and Celebrity Fight Night, patients receive not only the best available medical care, but a wealth of information and emotional support.

Contents

Part 1. Most Frequently Asked Questions   1

Questions 1–12 answer commonly asked questions regarding Parkinson disease, such as:
- What is Parkinson disease?
- What causes Parkinson disease?
- What are the stages of Parkinson disease?

Part 2. Tell Me More   37

Questions 13–27 discuss the symptoms and physical effects of Parkinson disease, as well as what to expect when you visit a neurologist:
- What are the main symptoms of Parkinson disease?
- Is difficulty speaking part of Parkinson disease?
- I am seeing a neurologist—what should I expect?
- What do I do after I've been diagnosed with Parkinson disease?

Part 3. Things You Should Know   89

Questions 28–38 review the progressive patterns of and physical changes brought on by Parkinson disease, including:
- Why does Parkinson disease get worse?
- What is freezing of gait?
- Why am I having difficulty swallowing?

Part 4. The First Five Years After You're Diagnosed   113

Questions 39–56 offer advice on what to expect during the first five years post diagnosis, including drug information and emotional changes, such as:
- What is the goal of treatment?
- What is a dopamine agonist?
- I have Parkinson disease—why me?
- As a care-partner, how can I cope with my partner's Parkinson disease?

I can think of no one better to write this book. If anyone knows the questions on the minds of patients with Parkinson disease, it is Dr. Abraham Lieberman.

This book will be a valuable resource. One could easily start at the beginning and go through it cover to cover. But it is just as valuable to open it at random and learn something new about Parkinson disease. The questions are organized along different topics, which is most valuable. The reader can quickly find the answer to a vexing question by searching for the topic in the table of contents and read about what is on his or her mind.

Dr. Lieberman has a gift of being able to communicate readily and with great facility. This ability comes across as one reads his answers to the questions posed in this book. This book is a marvelous addition to the literature on Parkinson disease and will be highly useful to those who want to learn what is on patients' minds and how to deal with these questions. Enjoy!

Stanley Fahn, MD
Scientific Director, Parkinson's Disease Foundation
Merritt Professor of Neurology,
Columbia University
New York, New York

Who is Abraham Lieberman?

If you have Parkinson disease, you may ask, who am I to write about it? I've studied PD for 40 years. I am the Director of the Muhammad Ali Parkinson Center charged with bringing educational and emotional support to all patients, caregivers, families, and friends of patients with Parkinson disease. I am also the Director of the Movement Disorder Clinic of the BNI, charged with diagnosing and evaluating people with PD and other movement disorders, teaching residents and fellows about PD and other movement disorders, and conducting research into PD and other movement disorders. The BNI is a world-renowned institute for neurology and neurosurgery. It is located on the campus of St. Joseph's Hospital in Phoenix, Arizona, which is consistently voted one of America's top hospitals.

I'm a 1959 graduate of Cornell University in Ithaca, New York; a 1963 graduate of the New York University School of Medicine; board certified in neurology and Psychiatry, and a fellow of the American Academy of Neurology, the American Neurological Association, and the Movement Disorder Society.

From July 1963 to June 1964, I interned at the Cincinnati General Hospital, part of the University of Cincinnati. From July 1964 until June 1967, I trained in neurology at Bellevue Hospital, one of the largest and busiest hospitals in America. During the Vietnam War, from 1967 to 1969, I was a neurologist at the United States Air Force Hospital in Tachikawa, Japan.

From 1970 to 1989, I was, successively, an instructor, an assistant professor, and a full professor of neurology at NYU. I was principal, or co-principal, investigator of more than 200 grants and studies on Alzheimer's disease, brain tumors, coma, depression, epilepsy, migraine headaches, nerve and muscle disease, Lewy Body disease, Parkinson disease, and stroke. Most of the studies involved devising ways of evaluating these diseases and developing treatments for them. The studies were contemplated by a large and varied neurology practice, seeing people who came from every corner of the globe to NYU to consult specialists in AIDS, cancer, cardiac surgery, endocrinology, GI disease, infectious disease, liver disease, neurosurgery, orthopedics, stroke, and psychiatry.

Beginning in 1970—but accelerating after 1980—my practice centered on Parkinson disease. My interest in Parkinson disease intensified in the nine years I spent as Director of Movement Disorders at the BNI in Phoenix (1989–1998). Here, with Muhammad and Lonnie Ali and Jimmy Walker, I helped start the Muhammad Ali Parkinson Center. In 1988, I moved to Miami to become the Harold S. Diamond Professor of Neurology at the University of Miami. In 2006, I left the University of Miami to start, with my wife Ina, the Lieberman Parkinson Clinic with offices in Miami Beach and Boca Raton. In Boca Raton, I worked with an outstanding group of physical, occupational, and speech therapists through Preferred Physical Therapy. Sheldon and Pam Devons, Trevor Meyerowitz, and Sue Levy broadened my understanding of the importance of physical, occupational, and speech therapy in maintaining patients at their best level of performance. Working closely with them, we developed many innovative therapies, some of which are discussed in this book. During this time, I answered questions from both my Web site and the Parkinson Research Foundation (PRF) Web site through the courtesy of Larry Hoffheimer, President of the PRF. In 2007, I was invited back to the BNI by my long-time friend, Dr. William Shapiro, Chairman of Neurology, and by Dr. Robert Spetzler, Chairman of Neurosurgery and Director of the BNI.

My interest in Parkinson disease was stimulated by a revolutionary breakthrough, the introduction of levodopa (L-dopa) by Dr. George Cotzias in 1967. That interest was sharpened at NYU by the presence of gifted scientists in biochemistry, neurochemistry, neuropharmacology, neurophysiology, and neuropsychology. I am especially indebted to Dr. Menek Goldstein, a renowned neurochemist, and Drs. Albert Goodgold and Julius Korein—renowned clinicians who introduced me to the great thinkers in Parkinson disease and made me critical of myself.

With colleagues at NYU, the University of Miami, and the BNI, I have authored or co-authored more than 200 articles published in major medical and neurology books and journals, including the *New England Journal of Medicine, Lancet, Journal of the American Medical Association, Annals of Internal Medicine, Annals of Neurology, Archives of Neurology, Journal of Neurology, Neurosurgery, and Psychiatry*, and *Journal of Pharmacology and Therapeutics*.

On a personal note, I have been married for 45 years to Ina Lieberman, a pediatric anesthesiologist and now my partner at the BNI Movement Disorder Clinic. We have four children, two daughters-in-law, two sons-in-law, and eight grandchildren. At age six, I had polio and spent 18 months in hospitals, clinics, and rehabilitation centers. Due to that experience, I know first-hand the anxiety, uncertainty, insecurity, fear, and panic centered around having a disease, both as a patient and now as a neurologist.

PART ONE

Most Frequently Asked Questions

What is Parkinson disease?

What causes Parkinson disease?

What are the stages of Parkinson disease?

More . . .

1. What is Parkinson disease?

Parkinson disease (PD) is a disease of the nervous system. Initially, PD affects a region of the brain called the basal ganglia, a region that regulates movement, posture, and balance. In time, PD may affect the cortex, the thinking and remembering part of the brain. And, in time, PD may affect the **autonomic nervous system** (ANS), which regulates blood pressure, the bowels and the bladder. All of these areas are affected by PD.

PD is, in part, a disease of slowed movement: everything you do takes longer. PD is also, in part, a disease of fast movement: the tremors of PD are 4 to 6 cycles per second (CPS)—faster than the eye can count. Why are some of the movements fast and others slow?

Willed, voluntary movement begins in the **cortex**, the thinking part of your brain. Your cortex specifies the speed, amplitude, direction, shape, regularity, and duration of each movement you make. The cortex is like the President, or chief executive, of your brain. Once your cortex decides on a course of movement, like walking down a road or up a flight of steps, it must decide how the movement will look (speed, amplitude, duration, etc.), then it "asks" the **basal ganglia** (a subconscious region of your brain) to set up rules that will govern these movements and allow them to go or stop in response to changing conditions, such as a bump in the road or a cat lying on the staircase. The basal ganglia are like Congress— they formulate the commands of the cortex into repetitive ongoing movements (e.g., walking) that continue while the cortex directs your attention to other things.

Just like Congress, the basal ganglia have two parts. The first includes the **substantia nigra**, which is like the "Go" party that wants to implement the President's commands. In PD, the substantia nigra is damaged,

Autonomic nervous system (ANS)

The portion of the brain and nervous system that governs or regulates the body's internal environment.

Cortex

The thinking part of the brain.

The cortex is like the President, or chief executive, of your brain.

Basal ganglia

A series of interconnected regions of the brain including the striatum, globus pallidus, and thalamus.

Substantia nigra

A portion of the brain with darkly pigmented cells that is a principal location affected by PD.

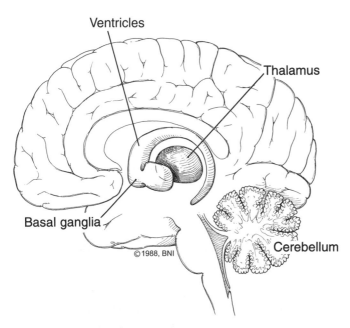

Ventricles

Thalamus

Basal ganglia

©1988, BNI

Cerebellum

Figure 1   Position of the cortex, ventricles, basal ganglia, thalamus, and cerebellum: the main "players" in PD.

Figure courtesy of Barrow Neurological Institute.

preventing the basal ganglia from correctly carrying out the cortex's commands, which results in slowed or incomplete movements. The basal ganglia also include the **globus pallidus** and the **subthalamic nucleus**, which function as modulators of the cortex's commands, or a "Stop" party. The interaction of the damaged "Go" and "Stop" parties results in various combinations of fast and slow movements.

The **cerebellum** (literally "little brain" in Latin) sits below the basal ganglia (see **Figure 1**). Damage to the cerebellum results in disorders of balance. Patients with disease of the cerebellum are unsteady and they may teeter or lurch as though they are drunk. The cerebellum is like the Supreme Court of the brain: it judges whether the movements being carried out by the basal ganglia (the Congress) are faithful to the commands of the cortex (the President). Even though the cerebellum is

Globus pallidus

A portion of the basal ganglia affected in PD. This region of the brain is known to be overactive in animal models of PD.

Subthalamic nucleus

An area of the brain located below the thalamus that acts as a "brake" on the substantia nigra.

Cerebellum

The coordinating center of the brain that acts as a "first responder" to information from the nervous system.

3

Cardinal symptoms

The four main symptoms of PD.

Resting tremor

A trembling of the hands or feet that occurs only when not in motion.

Rigidity

Stiffness or tightness of the muscles.

Bradykinesia

A primary symptom of PD that consists of slow movement, an incompleteness of movement, a difficulty in initiating movement, and an arrest of ongoing movement are associated with this slowness.

Postural instability

A lack of balance or unsteadiness while standing or changing positions.

Shaking Palsy

Paralysis agitans or trembling paralysis.

Paralysis Agitans

An agitated or trembling paralysis.

30% of all people with PD never have a tremor, and people with PD are not paralyzed.

undamaged in PD, it believes the basal ganglia are behaving incorrectly, and in trying to "correct" them, makes things worse by causing lurching or trembling.

2. How is Parkinson disease diagnosed?

Parkinson disease is diagnosed on the presence of two of the four main or **cardinal symptoms**. The cardinal symptoms include: a **resting tremor**, **rigidity** or stiffness, **bradykinesia** (defined as slowness and incompleteness of movement), and **postural instability** (defined as a loss of balance and difficulty walking). The disease is named for James Parkinson, an English doctor, who first described it in 1817.

Most people think of PD as a disease of trembling. Indeed it's been called the "**shaking palsy**" or "**paralysis agitans**" (an agitated or trembling paralysis). Yet, 30% of all people with PD never have a tremor, and people with PD are not paralyzed. The resting tremor of PD is different than the tremor of **essential tremor** (ET), a disease sometimes confused with PD. The tremor associated with ET increases when you stretch your hand, activating the muscles, and stops when you rest your hand. This type of tremor can be referred to as an action, sustention, or postural tremor, because you are sustaining a given posture of your hand by activating the muscles.

The tremor of ET can usually (but not always) be distinguished from the tremor of PD, as the ET tremor generally starts in both hands, while the PD tremor generally starts in one hand and spreads to the leg on the same side of the body before spreading to the other hand. Additionally, the tremor of PD may affect the chin, but rarely the head, while the tremor of ET rarely affects the chin. About 50% of people with ET have a family history of it, but only 15% of people with PD have a family history of PD. Sometimes PD can start with an action or sustention tremor, causing it to be mistaken for ET. As other PD symptoms evolve, it becomes apparent that PD is the correct diagnosis.

The rigidity, or stiffness, of PD affects the muscles of your neck, arms, and legs, and is usually greater on the same side of your body as the tremor. Sometimes the simultaneous occurrence of tremor and rigidity in an arm or leg gives a "ratchet-like" quality to the movement, like two gears meshing and moving in opposite directions. This phenomenon, known as "cog-wheeling," is diagnostic of PD only when associated with other symptoms.

The movement disorder of PD consists of slowness and incompleteness of movement referred to as bradykinesia. Although "brady" in Latin means slow and "kinesia" in Latin means movement, bradykinesia is more than slow movement. A turtle, when he walks, walks slowly, but the turtle is not bradykinetic. Each successive step of the turtle's legs is equally slow, and each successive step is equally small. When a person with PD walks, he walks slowly and each successive step may become slower and slower and shorter and shorter until he suddenly stops or "freezes." Or, occasionally, each successive step may become faster and faster until he runs, and often falls. The basal ganglia regulate these kinds of automatic movements (stepping movements made while walking) such that once started, they flow automatically without your conscious awareness of taking each step. In some ways, the actions of the basal ganglia are like those of a copy machine. Once you put in the "original" (the command to walk), the copies come automatically, each one resembling the original (each step like the next). In PD, the basal ganglia are

Essential tremor

A disease sometimes confused with PD.

like a defective copy machine; the first copy is as dark and readable as the original, but each succeeding copy grows lighter and lighter and less readable.

The postural instability, or balance problem, of PD may appear as an inability to stand on one leg, called "static balance." It may show up as losing your balance while turning or walking downstairs. When you turn or walk down a flight of stairs, for a split second you raise one leg off the ground, and at that moment, without your being aware that you raised your leg, you stumble and lose your balance. Postural instability may also show up as an inability to right or correct yourself when you stumble or are pushed, which is called "dynamic balance." Dynamic balance depends upon your brain's ability to receive "messages" from sensors in your feet that subconsciously monitor the position of your feet in space, as well as from sensors in your inner ears. Messages from the sensors in your feet and inner ears are relayed to a part of your brain called the **thalamus**. The loss of dynamic balance occurs because of a mismatch of the signals from your feet and inner ears, and the inability of your basal ganglia and spinal cord to adjust your muscles to a changing environment.

Thalamus

Portion of the brain that receives impulses from the nerves and transmits it to the conscious brain.

An important, but not cardinal, symptom is the stooped posture that occurs in up to 60% of people with PD. Stooping of the neck, or stooping or slumping of the shoulders and spine, may be early symptoms of PD (see **Figure 2**). The stooping may result from an uneven pull of the flexor muscles in front of the spine over the extensor muscles in back of the spine and it may be aggravated by osteoporosis. The significance of stooping is discussed later in this book.

In 1998, my colleagues and I developed the following test that can help you determine if you have PD.

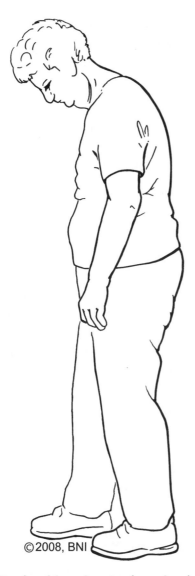

©2008, BNI

Figure 2   Stooping of the neck, or stooping or slumping of the shoulders and spine, may be early symptoms of PD.

Figure courtesy of Barrow Neurological Institute.

Self-Assessment Test for Parkinson Disease:

- Do you have trouble getting up from a chair?
- Has your handwriting become smaller?*
- Do people say your voice has become softer?

- Do your feet ever seem to get stuck to the floor?
- Do people say your face always seems sad?
- Do your hands or legs shake or tremble?
- Do you have difficulty buttoning buttons?
- Do you shuffle your feet when you walk?
- Do you take tiny steps when you walk?
- Has anyone asked if you have Parkinson disease?
- Have you ever taken levodopa/carbidopa or Sinemet?

Score one point for every "yes" answer.
Score 0–4: Low probability of PD
Score 5–9: Moderate probability of PD
Score 10–11: High probability of PD

*Samples of your handwriting obtained during a doctor's visit and compared with samples from the past several years (such as your signature on annual tax returns), may be used as an indicator of PD (see **Figure 3**). PD causes a condition called **micrographia**: when a patient's handwriting gets smaller and more compressed. You, as a patient, should write a sentence: "This is a sample

Micrographia

A PD symptom in which the affected individual's handwriting becomes small and illegible due to decreasing control over hand muscles.

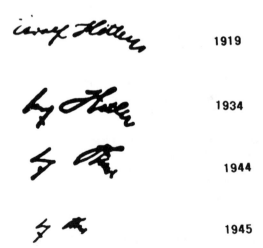

1919

1934

1944

1945

Figure 3   Samples of Adolf Hilter's handwriting shows progression of micrographia. The disease probably began in 1934. The signature appears to be normal until you compare it with the signature in 1919.

of my best handwriting" every day, first thing in the morning before taking any medication. Over the years, these handwriting samples can be a window into the progression or lack of progression of PD.

3. Is PD mainly a disease of older people?

Although PD is more common in older people, it is not exclusive to them. The peak onset of PD is 60 years, which is hardly considered old these days. Moreover, 15% of PD patients are younger than 50, and 10% are younger than 40.

In the United States, for every million people about 3,500 have PD; altogether there are about 1.2 million people with PD in the United States. Given that the development of symptoms is slow, the time between onset and diagnosis may be from 2 to 10 years. Due to the long period between the onset of the "process of PD" (which is usually silent) and diagnosis, it's estimated that for every person who's diagnosed with PD there are at least two or more who have PD but have not yet been diagnosed.

The reason age plays a role in the development of PD is that the slowness of movement and the rigidity of PD results from a loss of neurons (cells) in a region of the brain called the substantia nigra. As we age, we lose approximately 2,000 neurons a year. The "process of PD" results in an increased loss of neurons: 5,000 to 20,000 neurons per year. The older you are, the fewer neurons you have from the normal age-related loss of neurons, the more vulnerable you are to the accelerated loss of neurons in PD, and therefore the more likely you are to develop PD. The incidence of PD may increase as the overall population ages unless we find a way of stopping or slowing it down.

Although easily diagnosed when advanced, mild or early PD can be difficult to diagnose, especially in young people who, it's thought, are not as likely to get PD. Approximately 5.0% of people with PD have Young Onset Parkinson Disease (YOPD). YOPD is defined as onset at 40 years or younger. In the United States, there are approximately 50,000 people with YOPD. YOPD and PD are similar but different. Except for age of onset, YOPD in large part resembles adult onset PD. YOPD is thought to represent the lower end of the age spectrum for idiopathic, adult onset PD. In YOPD, as in adult PD, symptoms start insidiously and progress slowly over several years. YOPD is more likely to be genetic than older onset PD.

Tremor is often the most common initial symptom in YOPD, occurring in 70% of patients. In some patients it's present all the time, in others only during times of stress or fatigue. Tremor usually starts in the thumb or the wrist on one side of the body. Occasionally the tremor in YOPD may start in or involve the jaw. **Dystonia** (involuntary muscle spasms) is a common initial symptom in YOPD, but not in adult onset PD. Dystonia may appear as an aching pain in the shoulder or upper arm (where it's often mistaken for arthritis) or a cramping pain in a calf or foot (where it's often mistaken for a muscle ache related to sports).

4. What causes Parkinson Disease?

The main symptoms of Parkinson disease result from a lack of a chemical substance in the brain, a specific neuro-transmitter (so called because it transmits messages from one cell to another) called **dopamine**. In PD, dopamine is lacking in the region of the brain called the substantia nigra, as well as in the connections of the substantia nigra with another region called the **striatum**

Dystonia

Involuntary muscle spasms resulting in awkward and sustained postures, which may be painful. Dystonia can involve the eyes, neck, the trunk, and the limbs.

Dopamine

A chemical messenger in the brain; loss of dopamine is a key factor in PD.

Striatum

A portion of the brain, connected with the substantia nigra, which is affected by PD.

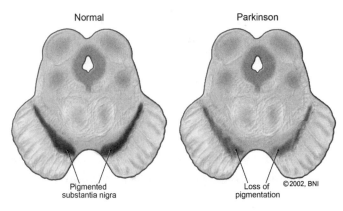

Figure 4   Relationship of the substantia nigra to the striatum.

Figure courtesy of Barrow Neurological Institute.

(See **Figure 4**). The substantia nigra contains darkly pigmented, black cells (its name means "black substance" in Latin). The cells targeted by PD contain one or more round bodies, called **Lewy bodies**, which in turn contain a protein called alpha synuclein. It is not yet known why the substantia nigra is targeted in PD.

Lewy bodies
Small, iridescent pinkish spheres found in the dying nerve cells of people with PD.

There are two types of neurons in the nigra, one type contains a protein called calmodulin, and the other does not. The calmodulin-containing neurons are the ones targeted. Among the theories proposed are: that the calmodulin neurons are genetically more vulnerable; that they are more susceptible to a number of toxins or viruses; that their membranes contain openings (or channels) that permit an increased entry of calcium and/or iron which damage the neurons; that the **mitochondria** (which act as the neurons' power-plants) are defective and do not generate enough energy to sustain the neurons; or that the mitochondria generate too many toxic products, called free radicals, and that these damage the neurons.

Mitochondria
Cellular energy sources.

Other theories propose that an enzyme in the mitochondria, called **monoamine oxidase B** (**MAO-B**), increases with age, resulting in an increased production of toxic free radicals. This has led to the use of MAO-B blockers (inhibitors), such as rasagiline (Azilect) and selegiline (Eldepryl, Zelapar) to slow the progression of PD. Still other theories propose that the neurons die because of a lack of specific growth or trophic factors including **glial derived neurotrophic factor** (GDNF) and **nurturin**.

Recently, researchers Braak and Del Tredici have proposed that PD does not begin in the substantia nigra; rather the earliest changes are in a region of the brainstem called the **dorsal vagal nucleus**. The dorsal vagal nucleus is the "head" or "chief" nucleus of the para-sympathetic nervous system (part of the autonomic nervous system, or ANS). The para-sympathetic nervous system is the "calming" part of the ANS and its involvement may be partly responsible for the increased anxiety and depression that occurs in patients with PD.

Following the dorsal vagal nucleus, another part of the brainstem, the **locus ceruleus**, is involved and may account in part for the sleep disturbances involved in PD. After the dorsal vagal nucleus and the locus ceruleus, the following neurons are involved: neurons of the olfactory cortex (the part of our brains responsible for sense of smell); neurons of the substantia nigra; and neurons of the amygdala and hypothalamus, the nuclei of the sympathetic part of the ANS, which controls our heart rate, heart contractility, blood pressure, rate and depth of breathing, and endocrine glands. Finally, the neurons of the hippocampus and the nucleus basalis (the memory banks of the brain), and the neurons of the cortex, are involved.

5. What puts me at risk for developing Parkinson disease?

The process of PD in your body may start 5 to 20 years before the first symptoms are recognized. In those rare cases of inherited PD, the process may even start at birth. The long period between the onset of the process of PD and the appearance of symptoms makes it difficult to distinguish those factors that may have caused the disease from those factors that may have sped up a disease that was incubating.

The process of PD in your body may start 5 to 20 years before the first symptoms are recognized.

The following factors are associated with an increased risk of developing PD. It's not known if each of these factors is a direct cause of PD or if it's an indirect cause that increases the susceptibility to developing PD:

- People 60 years or older
- People who have a family member with PD
- People exposed to toxic chemicals (the degree and duration of exposure are important, but are usually not known or documented)
- People who continuously and habitually use amphetamines, cocaine, heroin, and methamphetamine
- People who had encephalitis (a viral infection of the brain)
- People who had a significant brain injury
- People with Gaucher's disease (there is a link between the genetics of PD and the genetics of Gaucher's disease)

6. Is Parkinson disease inherited?

Heredity, or genetic predisposition, may play a role in developing PD. Between 15% and 25% of people with PD report that another relative also has PD. In about 1% of families, PD is known to occur in many members

Heredity

Genetic transmission from parent to child.

13

over several generations. Studies of the genetics of these families have identified specific, mutated **genes** that are linked to PD. However, the results cannot be generalized to all people with PD.

Genes are the basis for heredity. A gene consists of a long strand of four molecules (**DNA**) arranged like beads on the 23 pairs of **chromosomes** found in each of us. Each chromosome carries thousands of genes and each gene consists of thousands of molecules of DNA. Genes determine the way in which proteins, the "building blocks" of your body, are made. Hence, if a gene is abnormal, the protein it encodes will be abnormal, and some of these abnormal proteins may cause PD. So far, scientists have identified several mutations and several different locations in humans that are involved in PD. But there is much more to learn.

One of the first genes associated with PD, called alpha synuclein (also called Parkin 1), has been identified on chromosome 4 and is responsible for a relatively rare inherited form of PD. Alpha synuclein is found in Lewy bodies. It appears that the gene mutation involved in the production of alpha synuclein may start a biochemical cascade of events that eventually kills the cell. If the biochemical cascade leading to cell death, called apoptosis, can be interrupted by finding the right drug, a cure may be found.

A second gene, which is on chromosome 6, was found by Japanese researchers and is named the Parkin 2 gene. The Parkin 2 gene is found within the nucleus of cells and plays a role in "digesting" proteins. It appears that Parkin 2 gene essentially destroys defective or old proteins. If the Parkin 2 gene itself is defective, the process of destruction is slowed and the defective

Genes

Long strands of four molecules that determine the way in which proteins are made. Genes are the basis of heredity.

DNA

DNA, or deoxyribonucleic acid, is the hereditary material in humans and almost all other organisms.

Chromosomes

Collections of genes that compose DNA. All people have 23 pairs of chromosomes in every cell.

proteins increase, becoming toxic to the cell by oxidizing and releasing toxic **free radicals**, which damage the cell or the DNA contained within the cell. Researchers feel that interplay between several genes and several environmental toxins may be responsible for PD.

Genes encode proteins and, ultimately, proteins and how they interact with the environment are a major determinant of many diseases, including PD. An abnormally mutated protein is one factor that determines how that particular protein interacts with the internal and external environment of the cell. Although at present abnormal genes are the sole cause of PD in only one percent of patients with PD, it's anticipated that as our understanding of genetics grows, more abnormal genes, such as the LRRK 2 gene found in up to 5% of all patients with PD, including those without a family history of PD, will be found. Much attention is focused on the LRRK 2 gene because it appears in adults, not adolescents, with PD and of the interactions of the protein encoded by the LRRK 2 gene with environmental factors as a cause of PD.

7. Do toxins in the environment cause PD?

There are, literally, hundreds of thousands of potential toxins in the air, the soil, in your home, at your work, and in your food and water. Whether any given toxin causes PD has not yet been clinically proven. Effects of toxins, and the possibility of their causing PD-like symptoms, depends on chemical structure, concentration in the environment, duration of exposure (usually measured in months or years), the toxin's ability to penetrate your skin, nose, lungs or gut and reach your brain, its ability to attach itself to the pigmented neurons in your substantia nigra, and its ability to damage

Free radicals

Toxic molecules that arise from the breakdown and oxidation of foods and naturally occurring body chemicals.

Table 1   Summarizes the known information on the genes involved in PD, the chromosomes they are located on, the age of onset of PD, whether the inheritance is dominant or recessive, and the protein the gene encodes.

Gene	Chromosome	Onset (yrs)	Inherit	Protein
Park 1, 4	4	40s	Dominant	Alpha synuclein Messenger
Park 2	2	20s	Recessive	Parkin Chaperone
Park 3	2	60s	Dominant	Unknown
Park 5	4	50s	Dominant	UCHL1 Chaperone
Park 6	1	40s	Recessive	PINK 1, mitochondria Protein kinase
Park 7	1	40s	Recessive	DJ-1, increases dopamine, increases sensitivity DA receptor
Park 8	12	50s	Dominant	LRRK 2 leucine rich repeat kinase Dardarin
Park 10	1	60s	Dominant	Unknown
Park 11	2	60s	Dominant	Unknown

your DNA or the proteins in your cells. The toxin may act directly or through free radicals (an unstable atom or group of atoms that are highly reactive and capable of biological damage).

Each cell in your body has a limited ability to repair the damaged DNA, to "soak-up" the free radicals. The molecules that "soak-up" the free radicals are called **antioxidants**. Antioxidants work by offering easy electron targets for the free radicals, thus "trapping" the electron and making it stable. Each cell has only a limited quantity of antioxidants. While it has not been

Antioxidants

Substances that bind free radicals and prevent them from damaging cells.

proven that free radicals cause PD, or that increasing your intake of antioxidants prevents PD, a diet that includes antioxidant-rich foods, such as blueberries, cranberries, apples, and blackberries, will certainly increase your body's ability to fight off free radicals.

While antioxidants are needed to soak-up or inactivate free radicals, not all free radicals are bad. Determining which free radicals are good and under which conditions is a challenge; one being met by a better understanding of the cell and its naturally occurring antioxidants. One such naturally occurring antioxidant is the pigmented melanin granules in the substantia nigra, the granules that give the nigra, the "black substance," its name.

Some of the toxins that have been linked to PD or PD-like symptoms include:

- *Chlorine*—including chlorine used in bleaches, detergents, and swimming pools; methylene chloride used in pharmaceuticals, chemical processing, and aerosols; perchloroethylene and tricholoroethylene used in adhesives and cleaning; and polyvinyl chloride used in plastics.
- *Manganese*—including exposure from mining or welding.
- *Mercury*—used (in the past) in dental amalgams, fluorescent lamps, thermometers, and in the preservative Thimerosol in vaccines.
- *MPTP*—a chemical used in making animal models of PD.
- *Rotenone*—a pesticide used in making animal models of PD.

Even though mercury has been linked to PD-like symptoms, the amount of mercury given off from dental amalgams is small—not enough to make you sick.

The methyl mercury found in fish and other sea animals (clams, oysters, snails), is also not enough to make you sick. It is possible that the cumulative effect of mercury in one's system could cause neurological symptoms; however, there is no proof that mercury in humans or animals causes PD.

Likewise, increased iron in the brain has been linked to PD. Interestingly, while the normal brain contains 50 mg of iron; the Parkinson brain contains five times as much iron: 250 mg. Iron helps several enzymes involved in DNA and protein synthesis and repair. Although there is no proof at this time that the increased iron in the substantia nigra is a cause of PD, many investigators are trying to develop drugs, **chelators**, which detoxify and remove metal ions from the brain. The goal of iron chelation in the brain is to prevent any iron-mediated injury to the neurons. The MAO-B inhibitor, rasagiline is, in part, an iron chelator and some believe this may be partly responsible for their usefulness.

Finally, some people wonder if **manganese fumes** from welding can cause PD. Manganese poisoning can result from exposure to manganese dust and vapors, such as occurs in certain miners and welders, and from the ingestion of food that is contaminated with manganese. Manganese, when inhaled or ingested, is excreted through the kidney and feces, as well as through saliva, perspiration, and the lungs. Once manganese is absorbed, its distribution depends upon its transformation, its binding to the body's proteins, and its entry into the brain. **Welding**, the process of joining metals together using a filler and an electric arc, produces fumes and gases that contain a number of elements, including manganese. Welding may cause upper respiratory symptoms, pulmonary edema (water

Chelators
Drugs which detoxify and remove metal ions from the brain.

Manganese fumes
Fumes generated in the process of welding that some believe may cause PD.

Some people wonder if manganese fumes from welding can cause PD.

Welding
The process of joining metals together using a filler and an electric arc.

on the lung), pulmonary fibrosis (scarring of the lung) and lung cancer. Welding has also been associated with bladder and throat cancers. Neurologic complications include confusion and delusions from the fumes (called "fume fever").

Parkinson symptoms have been described in both miners and welders. Although manganese miners are known to develop PD symptoms from inhalation of manganese dust or ingestion of food contaminated with manganese, it's unclear whether this also happens in welders. At Washington University in St. Louis, a study compared the features of PD in 15 career welders to control groups with PD. Researchers found that welders had a younger age at onset (46 years) of PD compared with controls (63 years). There was no difference in frequency of tremor, slowness of movement, rigidity, postural instability, family history, clinical depression, or dementia. All treated welders responded to levodopa. Motor fluctuations and dyskinesias occurred at a similar frequency in welders and the control group. PET scans with 6-flurodopa obtained in several welders showed findings typical of PD. This suggests, but does not prove, that welding causes a PD-like disorder. There is a strong disagreement as to whether welding causes PD. Most experts believe welding does not cause PD. As post-mortem studies have not been done on welders, it is not known if the pathology of PD in welders is similar to or different from true PD.

Agent Orange is the name of herbicide developed for the military, primarily for use as a defoliant to destroy enemy cover during the Vietnam War (1964–1972), and is thought by some to cause PD. Agent Orange is a 50-50 mix of two chemicals, including **tetrachlorodibenzodioxin (TCDD)**, which were mixed with kerosene

Agent Orange

A herbicide developed for the military and thought by some to cause PD.

Tetrachlorodibenzodioxin (TCDD)

Prototype for a class of halogenated aromatic hydrocarbons, which appear to have a common mechanism of action and to produce similar effects, although they differ in potency; achieved notoriety in the 1970s when it was discovered to be a contaminant in the herbicide Agent Orange and was shown to produce birth defects in rodents.

19

or diesel fuel and dispersed by aircraft. An estimated 19 million gallons of Agent Orange were used in Vietnam during the war. Part of the concern about Agent Orange was about its contamination with dioxin. Dioxins are found in nature and are related to toxins that may cause cancer. In laboratory tests on animals, dioxin causes several diseases but not, to date, PD. The other concern about Agent Orange regards TCDD and how it affects the brain. Veterans who served in the military during the Vietnam War are now at an age range when PD occurs and many claim their PD is related to Agent Orange. However, it is not known if there's a higher prevalence of PD among veterans who were exposed to Agent Orange versus age-matched controls. Likewise, it is not known if there's a higher prevalence of PD among Vietnamese who were exposed to Agent Orange versus age-matched controls. Furthermore, individual veterans had different levels of exposure depending on their military tasks. The likelihood is that, barring new developments, the role of Agent Orange in causing PD will stay unresolved.

Some people wonder if drugs, either prescription or non-prescription, can cause PD. What the medical community has found is that PD symptoms, not true PD, can be caused by drugs, and these symptoms are reversible upon stopping the drug. In contrast, true PD is an irreversible disease. Occasionally a person with unrecognized PD is "unmasked" by taking drugs; the person's PD would have appeared eventually, but it appeared sooner because of the drug. Drugs known to cause PD symptoms include haldol, mellaril, prolixin, stellazine, and thorazine. Called **major tranquillizers** (also known as **neuroleptics**), these were the first drugs successfully used to treat the symptoms of psychosis and schizophrenia. Other drugs causing PD symptoms

Neuroleptics

The first drugs successfully used to treat the symptoms of psychosis and schizophrenia (also called major tranquillizers).

include orap, risperidal, trilafon, and zyprexa. These are newer drugs, and they have been used to successfully treat the symptoms of bi-polar disorder, obsessive-compulsive disorder, psychosis, and schizophrenia. As a rule, they are less likely to cause PD symptoms than haldol, prolixin, stellazine, and thorazine. Not all medications that cause PD symptoms treat psychiatric problems; compazine and reglan, drugs used to treat nausea, vomiting, and acid reflux, may also cause such symptoms. These drugs all have in common an ability to fully or partly block dopamine receptors in the brain. In effect, they cause PD symptoms by making the receptors unavailable to the brain's own dopamine. Drugs known to cause PD symptoms also include reserpine (a drug once used to lower blood pressure) and tetrabenazine (used to control dyskinesia, a condition described later). These two drugs deplete the brain of dopamine. This depletion is temporary and levels return to normal after the drugs are stopped.

The prevalence of PD symptoms in people taking these prescription drugs varies from 15–60% and depends on the drug, the dose, time on the drug, the person's age (older people are more susceptible), and the person's sensitivity; some people are more likely to develop PD symptoms than others. Usually, PD symptoms appear weeks or months after the drug is started (rarely sooner) and disappear weeks or months after the drug is stopped. The symptoms of drug-caused PD are almost indistinguishable from true PD; however there are two differences:

1. Drug-induced PD symptoms appear on both sides of the body at the same time. The symptoms of true PD appear first on one side of the body, and later on the other side.

Tardive

Movements in drug-induced PD that appear after the drug is started, or sometimes after the drug is stopped.

Dyskinesia

Dance-like involuntary movements. Dyskinesia may involve the face, the tongue, the head and neck, the trunk, the arms and legs.

Illegal drugs such as amphet-amines, cocaine, and metham-phetamine all deplete dopamine from stores in the brain and could, with chronic use, result in PD symptoms.

MPTP

A narcotic-like drug known to cause permanent PD symptoms.

2. The "pill-rolling," resting tremor of PD is less common in drug-caused PD symptoms. An action tremor, one that appears when the hands are moving and one faster than the pill-rolling tremor, is characteristic of drug-caused PD symptoms.

It's not known whether drug-caused PD symptoms are a "predictor" of the later development of PD. Drug-caused PD symptoms may be associated with dyskinesia—dance-like involuntary movements. Dyskinesia may involve the face, tongue, head and neck, trunk, arms and legs. The movements are called **tardive** (meaning delayed) **dyskinesia** because they appear after the drug is started, or sometimes after the drug is stopped. Although drug-caused PD symptoms and tardive dyskinesia are likely mediated by different mechanisms, the two may coexist in the same person. This combination presents a challenge because the treatment of one may aggravate the other.

In another category are drugs that cause permanent PD symptoms. Illegal drugs such as amphetamines, cocaine, and methamphetamine all deplete dopamine from stores in the brain and could, with chronic use, result in PD symptoms. The most notorious example of a drug that caused PD, and later became a means of creating an animal model of PD, is the drug abbreviated **MPTP**, a narcotic-like drug, the actions of which were described by Dr. J. William Langston. In his book, *The Case of the Frozen Addict*, Langston describes how a young heroin addict, George Carillo, unknowingly injected himself with heroin that had been contaminated with MPTP. Over several days George became increasingly paralyzed and even lost the ability to talk. Medical personal at a county hospital ER were unable to find a cause or cure and after many inconclusive tests, he was sent to a special hospital unit. In the hospital, George was diagnosed by Dr. Langston as having PD. Later, it was determined that George and several other addicts had developed PD as a result of injecting themselves with heroin contaminated with MPTP. MPTP was later shown by Dr. Langston (now at the California Parkinson Institute) and Dr. Stanley Burns (now at the Barrow Neurological Institute) to act as a "guided missile," specifically destroying nerve cells in the substantia nigra, the same nerve cells destroyed by the process that causes PD.

The difference between MPTP-related PD and true PD is that, in true PD, the dying cells contain a round structure called a Lewy body (see **Figure 5**), but this is absent in MPTP-caused PD. The Lewy body tells us something about what causes PD, but as yet researchers have not figured out exactly what it is. MPTP has served as an excellent means of causing PD in animals, which has provided researchers with insights into how PD may start and progress. It has also helped in the development of new drugs for PD.

8. Can a head injury or boxing cause Parkinson disease?

A small number of people (about 1%) who sustain a significant head injury later develop PD. A "significant head injury" means the person was in a coma for at least an hour, was hospitalized, and may have had surgery to remove a blood clot. The clot may have increased pressure inside the skull, causing downward pressure on the substantia nigra and this resulted in the death of enough nigral neurons to cause PD. A minor head injury, however, does not result in PD. A minor head injury is one that either doesn't result in a

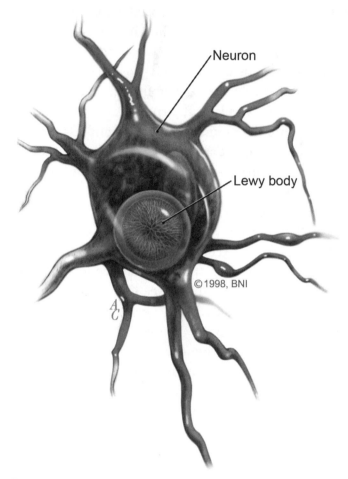

Figure 5   Dopamine nerve cell with Lewy body.
Figure courtesy of Barrow Neurological Institute.

loss of consciousness or results in only a brief loss of consciousness.

Due to the attention that has been called to one of the greatest boxers of all time, Muhammad Ali, and his struggle with PD, many people wonder if boxing causes PD. The repeated blows to the brain that boxers endure over several years can result in a condition called **dementia pugilistica**. The author has examined several boxers who suffer from dementia pugilistica,

Dementia pugilistica

A condition caused by repeated blows to the brain that some boxers develop over several years.

but Muhammad Ali does not have dementia pugilistica—he has typical PD. Muhammad Ali's PD began with a resting tremor of his left hand and later developed into a slowness of his hand and a shuffling gait, all of which are typical of PD. Muhammad Ali's PD has evolved slowly, over 22 years, unlike the evolution of dementia pugilistica, which rapidly progresses to dementia and inability to walk over the course of 5 years. By contrast, Muhammad Ali's mind is still sharp—he is not demented—and after 22 years with PD, he is still able to walk. Finally, the MRIs of boxers with dementia pugilistica show evidence of brain damage, while Muhammad Ali's MRIs do not.

In several studies, 15–40% of professional ex-boxers developed symptoms of Alzheimer's disease. At one end of the spectrum of ex-professional boxers is George Forman, who fought longer and suffered more blows to his head than Muhammad Ali, yet shows no signs of dementia. At the other end of the spectrum are severely affected ex-boxers who suffer from dementia pugilistica and are referred to as "punch drunk." In between are boxers with varying degrees of speech difficulty, rigidity, unsteadiness, memory loss, and inappropriate behavior. Symptoms, when they occur, usually begin shortly after the end of a boxer's career. On occasion they are first noticed after a hard bout. Symptoms in boxers develop an average of 16 years after they start to fight, although sometimes symptoms occur as early as 6 years into their boxing careers. Although symptoms occur in amateurs, they are more common in professionals. They occur in all weight classes, but are more common in heavyweights. Although the mechanism by which multiple and repeated blows to the head cause brain damage is not established, it is thought that such blows result in shearing injuries and multiple small hemorrhages. As the damage accumulates, minimal symptoms merge gradually into more obvious ones.

Autopsy examination of the brains of boxers with dementia pugilistica do not reveal the changes of PD (a loss of dopamine cells in the substantia nigra with the formation of Lewy bodies), but rather a loss of cells in the frontal and temporal lobes of the brain, as well as the amygdala (the "rage center") and the nucleus basalis. Less common are changes in the basal ganglia and the thalamus. The microscopic changes resemble those of Alzheimer's disease and include protein deposits around blood vessels (called amyloid plaques), and neurofibrillary tangles (twisted fibers of a tau protein inside the neurons) in the dying brain cells. The formation of Lewy bodies is not a part of dementia pugilistica.

9. Do strokes cause Parkinson disease?

Major strokes are caused by a blockage of large or medium-sized arteries: the "pipes" through which blood flows. Arteries harden in older people, especially if they have diabetes, high blood pressure, high cholesterol, or have smoked. If a large or medium-sized artery closes and if there are no arteries in the neighborhood that can replace it, the region of the brain the artery supplies is **infarcted**, meaning it dies. Unlike in PD where symptoms appear gradually and progress slowly over years, stroke symptoms appear suddenly and do not progress. The onset of PD is not dramatic; a selected group of neurons gradually die. A stroke is like a hurricane blowing away your house, while PD is more like a slow, steady rain eroding your basement.

Knowing the terminology used with strokes can be helpful. **Atherosclerosis** is the narrowing of a large

Unlike in PD where symptoms appear gradually and progress slowly over years, stroke symptoms appear suddenly and do not progress.

Infarcted

Death of a region of the brain supplied by a blocked artery.

Atherosclerosis

The narrowing of a large artery by cholesterol.

artery by cholesterol. Low cholesterol diets, the use of "statins" (drugs that lower cholesterol), exercise, anti-hypertensive drugs, and cessation of smoking are factors in fighting atherosclerosis. **Arteriosclerosis** is the narrowing of medium and small-sized arteries by cholesterol and by changes in the artery's muscular wall. The same factors that fight atherosclerosis will likewise fight arteriosclerosis. **Hypertension** (high blood pressure) contributes to and promotes both atherosclerosis and arteriosclerosis. Hypertension also results in the closure of tiny arteries, called arterioles. Such closure results in small infarctions known as lacunes, which individually cause no symptoms, but cumulatively may cause a variety of symptoms that mimic PD, especially when the lacunes occur in the basal ganglia (see **Figure 6**).

A single stroke does not cause PD. However, multiple "silent" or "minor" strokes affecting the striatum, globus pallidus, thalamus, cerebellum, and midbrain—regions that regulate balance, movement and walking—

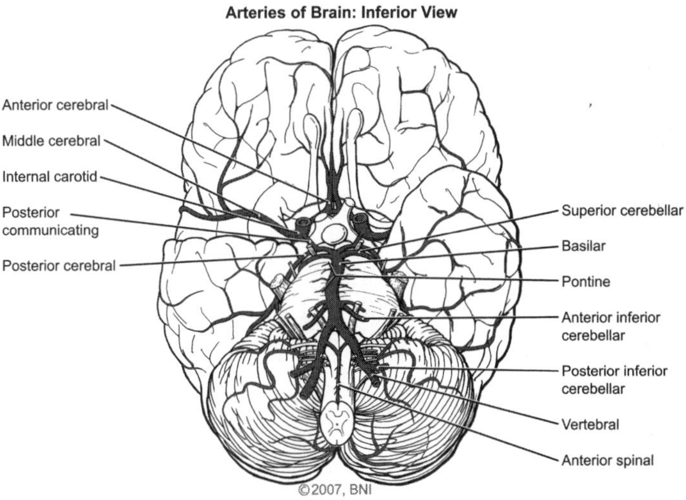

Arteriosclerosis

The narrowing of medium and small-sized arteries by cholesterol and by changes in the artery's muscular wall.

Hypertension

High blood pressure.

Arteries of Brain: Inferior View

Anterior cerebral
Middle cerebral
Internal carotid
Posterior communicating
Posterior cerebral

Superior cerebellar
Basilar
Pontine
Anterior inferior cerebellar
Posterior inferior cerebellar
Vertebral
Anterior spinal

©2007, BNI

Figure 6   Blood supply to the brain.
Figure courtesy of Barrow Neurological Institute.

Vascular Parkinson

Condition caused by a cumulative effect of multiple "silent" or "minor" strokes affecting the striatum, globus pallidus, thalamus, cerebellum, and midbrain that cause symptoms similar to PD.

Encephalitis lethargica

The sleeping sickness that occurred early in the 20th century with some symptoms resembling PD.

von Economo's encephalitis

See Encephalitis lethargica.

Parkinsonism

A class of movement disorders with similar symptoms. Parkinson disease is one of these disorders.

Epidemic delirium

One of the diagnoses for the mysterious "sleeping sickness" pandemic of the early 1900s (see von Economo's Encephalitis).

Epidemic schizophrenia

One of the diagnoses for the mysterious "sleeping sickness" pandemic of the early 1900s (see von Economo's Encephalitis).

may have a cumulative effect over several months or years that cause symptoms similar to PD. This condition is called **vascular Parkinson**, but the symptoms of vascular Parkinson usually do not respond to PD drugs. The treatment goal of vascular Parkinson is to prevent additional strokes. The course of the disease can be favorably altered by paying close attention to the factors that cause stroke.

Usually a neurologist or a PD expert can separate the effects of multiple minor strokes from those of PD, and those strokes can usually be seen on an MRI (magnetic resonance imaging) scan. Sometimes strokes and PD coexist; having PD does not protect you from having strokes, and vice-versa. How many of your symptoms are caused by stroke and how many by PD is likely something only a specialist trained in PD can determine.

10. Do viruses cause Parkinson disease?

Viruses have been suspected as a cause of PD since an epidemic of **"sleeping sickness"** (also called **encephalitis lethargica** or **von Economo's encephalitis**) occurred early in the 20th century. The following description of the epidemic and the **Parkinsonism** that followed it (post-encephalitic Parkinsonism) is found in Oliver Sack's book *Awakenings* (Harper Collins Books).

In the winter of 1916–1917 in Vienna and other cities, a "new" illness suddenly appeared, and rapidly spread over the next three years to become world-wide in its distribution. Manifestations of the sleeping sickness were so varied that no two patients ever presented exactly the same picture, and so strange as to call forth from physicians such diagnoses as **epidemic delirium, epidemic schizophrenia, atypical** *poliomyelitis*, etc. It seemed, at first, that a thousand new diseases had suddenly broken loose, and it was only through the profound clinical acumen of Constantin von Economo, allied with his pathological studies on the brains of patients who had died, and his demonstration that these, besides showing a unique pattern of damage, contained a virus which could transmit the disease to monkeys, that the identity of this protean disease was established.

In the ten years that it raged, this pandemic took or ravaged the lives of nearly five million people before it disappeared in 1927. A third of those affected died in the acute stages of the sleeping sickness; in states of coma so deep as to preclude arousal or in states of sleeplessness so intense as to preclude sedation.

Patients who suffered but survived an extremely severe somnolent-insomniac attack of this kind often failed to recover their original aliveness. They would be conscious and aware, yet not fully awake, they would sit motionless and speechless all day in their chairs, totally lacking energy, impetus, initiative, motive, appetite, affect or desire. They registered what went on about them without active attention and with profound indifference. They neither conveyed nor felt the feeling of life. They were as insubstantial as ghosts and as passive as zombies. Von Economo compared them to extinct volcanoes.

Atypical poliomyelitis

One of the diagnoses for the mysterious "sleeping sickness" pandemic of the early 1900s (see von Economo's Encephalitis).

Although no virus comparable to that of 1917–1927 has emerged, some experts believe PD could be related to a virus, one that invades the brain and changes the genetic composition of the affected neurons. Uncommon viruses, such as Japanese B, eastern and western equine encephalitis, and St. Louis encephalitis have been linked to PD. In addition, such common viruses as the influenza virus and possibly the West Nile virus *could* be linked to PD. The appeal of a viral cause of PD is that it would assume the virus, like the virus that caused von Economo's encephalitis, invaded the brain, caused symptoms, and after a long latent period—years after the initial symptoms had subsided or disappeared—was responsible for the appearance of PD symptoms. Similar to the theoretical viral model of PD is the actual model of post-polio syndrome, which this author has developed.

11. What are the stages of Parkinson disease?

In 1967, Drs. Margaret Hoehn and Melvin Yahr devised a 6-point scale from 0 to 5, in order to classify the stages of PD. When this scale was first created, levodopa had not yet changed the course of PD treatment, nor were dopamine agonists or MAO-B inhibitors prescribed. At the time, doctors might differ over which of two close stages a patient was in (Stage 1 vs. Stage 2), but not over a greater disparity, such as Stage 1 vs. Stage 3. Reasonable predictions could be made and thus a patient diagnosed as Stage 1 or Stage 2 might expect to progress to Stage 3 in 5–10 years, and Stage 4 in another 5–10 years. After 10–20 years most patients were significantly disabled and few survived 20 or more years.

Today, to rate the true stage of PD, patients would have to stop taking their PD drugs for at least one month. With the drugs "washed out" of their system, the underlying stage of PD would appear. However, for most patients such a "wash-out" or "drug holiday" is not practical or feasible. In the past, when there were few ways to counteract the adverse effects of levodopa, "drug holidays" were recommended to give patients a break from taking their medication. These drug holidays were poorly tolerated by patients: they became immobile; markedly depressed or anxious; developed difficulty swallowing and breathing; developed pneumonia; and occasionally developed a life-threatening disorder called neuroleptic malignant syndrome.

Aside from the impracticality of patients taking a drug holiday to reveal the underlying PD stage, making predictions about the progression of PD based on the Hoehn and Yahr Scale is further complicated by fluctuations in patient medication response. After 2–5 years, many patients fluctuate such that their days consist of being "**on**" (levodopa is working) followed by being "**off**" (levodopa not working). When this occurs, the patient is rated during both the "on" and "off" states, with the off state being a better measure of the underlying PD stage. Additionally, the Hoehn and Yahr Scale rates mobility, but does not rate anxiety, aberrant behavior, depression, dyskinesia, memory loss, difficulty thinking, or difficulty swallowing, all of which may overshadow a patient's lack of mobility.

On-off

In PD, the condition of alternating "on" (asymptomatic) periods with "off" periods in which symptoms such as freezing or dyskinesia are evident.

The Hoehn and Yahr Scale is *not* a cancer rating scale—it is not a guide to treatment and it is an imperfect guide to prognosis. When a person has cancer, a surgeon can stage a patient based on the type of cancer diagnosed and how far it has spread. This data, coupled with historical data on thousands of similar cancers, is then used to predict prognosis and survival. Similar data is not available for PD.

Progression of PD is related to how long you have had it, which is not the same as how long you have been diagnosed with it. The process of PD may have begun years earlier with the appearance of symptoms such as anxiety, depression, or anosmia (loss of smell). About 5% of patients will recall that 3–5 years prior to diagnosis of PD, even before initial symptoms became apparent, a mild symptom, such as a hand or foot turning in or a tremor of one hand appeared during a particularly stressful event. In addition to the traditional symptoms of PD (tremor, rigidity, slowness of movement, difficulty

Progression of PD is related to how long you have had it, which is not the same as how long you have been diagnosed with it.

walking), many PD patients develop a curved spine. Initially their chin touches their chest, then their shoulders stoop, and eventually their spine curves—either bending forward or to one side. A curved spine may, in fact, be the earliest symptom of PD. The curved spine of PD differs from the curved spine of osteoporosis in that with osteoporosis the curvature results from softening of the bones, while in PD the curve may result from an unequal pull of muscles; the muscles in front pulling harder than those in the back.

The progression of PD is related to a loss of cells in a region of the brain called the substantia nigra. Everyone is born with approximately 400,000 of these cells (neurons); 200,000 on each side of the brain. It is estimated that each year every one of us loses 2,000 of these neurons. When a person has cumulatively lost approximately 240,000 neurons, or 60%, the first symptoms of PD appear. Thus, if we all lived for 120 years, we would all likely have PD. It is thought that the process of PD (which begins before the first symptoms appear) is characterized by an increased rate in the destruction of neurons, perhaps up to 5, 10, or even 20 thousand a year. When PD begins in an older person—70 years or older—they have already lost at least 140,000 neurons simply through age-related attrition. The additional accelerated loss of neurons in PD results in a more rapid rate of progression of PD in older people.

The response of a patient to PD drugs probably affects the perception of the rate of PD progression. Therefore, a person whose medication successfully alleviates the symptoms of PD after several weeks generally has a better prognosis and outlook than a patient who either continues to have symptoms of PD while on medication or is troubled by its side effects.

Table 2   The Hoehn and Yahr Scale (modified)

Stage	Description	Notes
Stage 0	• No visible symptoms of PD	
Stage 1	• Symptoms of PD confined to one side of the body	
Stage 2	• Symptoms on both sides of the body • No difficulty walking	The average duration of Stages 0 to 2 in patients with age of onset between 51 to 69 years, is about 4 years, without PD drugs. With skilled use of PD drugs the average duration of Stages 0 to 2 is about 8 years.
Stage 3	• Symptoms on both sides of the body • Minimal difficulty walking	The average duration of Stage 3 in patients with age of onset between 51 to 69 years, with skilled use of PD drugs, is about four years.
Stage 4	• Symptoms on both sides of the body • Moderate difficulty walking	
Stage 5	• Symptoms on both sides of the body • Unable to walk	Predictions on the average duration of Stage 4 to 5 are less reliable because symptoms such as dementia, psychosis (delusions, hallucinations related to PD drugs), dyskinesia, falls, and difficulty with balance may play a major role, a role not reflected by the Stage which only measures movement.

While a number of other rating scales are presently available, the Hoehn and Yahr scale continues to be the simplest and most widely used (see **Table 2**). The scale classifies PD into five categories, from early, one-sided effects, to full disability. In staging the patient, a doctor notes whether the patient's Sinemet is working (and thus the patient is "on") or if it is not working and the patient is considered "off."

12. Can I die from Parkinson Disease?

In 1967, before effective drugs (such as levodopa, Mirapex, or Comtan) became available for PD, people diagnosed with PD lived, on average, 6–15 years from diagnosis to death. Some people with PD fell and fractured their hip, pelvis, or spine and were confined to bed. Other patients became immobile and were also confined to bed. For these patients, death came due to the complications of being bedbound. For example:

1. Some patients developed difficulty swallowing and they gagged or choked on their food, even when fed carefully. Their food was then aspirated or swallowed into the lungs, causing pneumonia. The rigidity of PD-restricted movement of the chest wall muscles created difficulty in inhaling and exhaling deeply, which is essential for overcoming pneumonia. As the pneumonia spread, the infection overwhelmed the body's defenses despite the use of antibiotics. Breathing became labored, oxygen levels fell, and the patients died. Sometimes the infection spread from the lungs to the blood, heart, liver, and kidneys, causing patients to die of blood poisoning, known as **sepsis**.

2. Other patients who were not turned in bed every hour and did not have one-to-one skilled nursing care developed pressure sores on their buttocks and lower back. The sores often became infected and the patients died from the infection.

3. For some patients, just lying in bed with their legs rigid and unmoving caused them to develop blood

Sepsis
Blood poisoning.

clots in their legs. The clots broke apart and spread to the lungs, effectively shutting them down and making the patients unable to breathe.

The introduction of effective medications, such as L-dopa, Comtan, Mirapex, Requip, and Neupro, has changed the dynamics of this disease. People diagnosed with PD now live on average 15–30 years from diagnosis to death. The drugs postpone the day when people become confined to bed, and this, in turn, postpones the complications of being bed-bound. Furthermore, antibiotics have improved, special stockings can reduce blood clots from forming in the legs, and anticoagulants (blood thinners) can reduce the chances of blood clots breaking apart and traveling to the lungs.

Do people die of PD? Technically not. But PD sets the body up for death. Whether patients die of PD, or from PD complications, they die. The remedy is research to find the cause of PD or slow its progression so patients can outlive its consequences. Many PD patients confronted with a disease that progresses feel helpless. They should not! They must not! There are 4 simple rules I try to teach patients:

The introduction of effective medications, such as L-dopa, Comtan, Mirapex, Requip, and Permax, has changed the dynamics of this disease. People diagnosed with PD now live on average 15-30 years from diagnosis to death.

1. "**P**" find a **PHYSICIAN** who understands PD, a physician to whom you can relate, who is concerned about you, and who is readily accessible. Parkinson disease is with you the rest of your life, and so is your physician.

2. "**A**" have a positive **ATTITUDE**. If you're depressed and unable to cope, your depression will likely deepen. Parkinson will defeat you if you let it.

3. **"R" REGULAR**. Take your medication as prescribed and establish a regular routine for physical therapy. You may not be able to exercise your way out of PD, but if you don't exercise, and exercise appropriately, PD will defeat you.

4. **"K" KNOWLEDGE**. Learn all you can about Parkinson disease. Initially it may overwhelm you, but knowledge is power and you need to know all you can about the disease with which you have been diagnosed.

PART TWO

Tell Me More

What are the main symptoms of Parkinson Disease?

Is difficulty speaking part of PD?

I am seeing a neurologist—what should I expect?

What do I do after I've been diagnosed with Parkinson disease?

More . . .

13. What are the main symptoms of PD?

There are four main, or primary, symptoms of PD. To diagnose PD, at least two of these symptoms must be present.

Tremor is the most characteristic symptom of PD and may be the first symptom in up to 70% of patients. It appears as a "beating" or oscillating movement, usually of the hands and occasionally of the feet or chin. The movement is regular (4–6 beats per second) and is rhythmic, with each movement resembling the other. The tremor usually appears when the muscles of the hands or feet are relaxed or at rest, hence the name **resting tremor**. The tremor usually, but not always, decreases or disappears when the muscles of the hands or feet contract during movement. The resting tremor of PD usually begins on one side of the body and later spreads either to the leg or to the other arm. The thumb is usually involved early and prominently. The tremor looks like you are rolling a cigar, coin, or pill between your thumb and index finger—hence the name "**pill-rolling**" **tremor**.

In 20% of people with PD, the tremor is also present or only present during movement. Tremors are usually named for their most prominent component and are categorized as **sustention** or **postural tremors** (present when sustaining a posture of your arms or body produces the tremor), **action** or **kinetic tremors** (present when you move your hands), or **intention tremors** (appearing or exaggerated as you reach for a specific object). Postural, action and intention tremors are usually prominent in another disorder, essential tremor, which may sometimes be confused with PD and is discussed further in Question 24.

Tremor

Involuntary trembling, usually of the hands or head.

Tremor is the most characteristic symptom of PD and may be the first symptom in up to 70% of patients.

Resting tremor

A trembling of the hands or feet that occurs only when not in motion.

"Pill-rolling" tremor

PD symptom that looks like rolling a cigar, coin, or pill between thumb and index finger.

Sustention or postural tremors

Tremor present when the limbs or trunk are kept in certain positions and when they are moved actively.

Kinetic tremor

Tremor that is present when you move your hands

Intention tremors

Tremors appearing or exaggerated as you reach for a specific object.

Rigidity in PD is described as stiffness or tightness of the muscles. Normally muscles contract and tighten when they move and relax or soften when at rest. In rigidity, the muscles of your arm or leg stay contracted and stretching them becomes difficult. Because of rigidity, your arm may not swing when you walk. The mask-like or expressionless face that characterizes PD also results, in part, from rigidity of your facial muscles. Some people with PD have "**cogwheel rigidity**" in which an arm or a leg "catches" during movement, resembling the way a cog catches in a wheel. The small, illegible, compressed handwriting (called micrographia) and the decreased eye blink of people with PD are also related, in part, to rigidity.

Cogwheel rigidity

PD symptom in which an arm or a leg "catches" during movement, resembling the way a cog catches in a wheel.

Bradykinesia means slow (brady) movement (kinesia). In addition to slow movement, bradykinesia includes an incompleteness of movement, a difficulty in initiating movement, and an arrest of ongoing movement. The incompleteness of movement is as important as the slowness of movement. Bradykinesia is the most prominent, and usually the most disabling, symptom of PD. With bradykinesia, you may have difficulty walking, as well as difficulty speaking, swallowing and turning.

Postural instability is a lack of balance or unsteadiness while standing or changing positions. The postural instability of standing or balancing yourself on one foot (called **static balance**) involves different mechanisms than the postural instability of changing positions, such as when you're turning or pivoting, which is called **dynamic balance**. Some of the things that you did automatically, such as "righting" or correcting yourself after being bumped or pushed, become difficult and you may fall. The postural reflexes that initiate the corrective movements are located deep in the brain and are affected in PD.

Static balance

Balance in which the body maintains equilibrium for one position.

Dynamic balance

The ability to right yourself when stumbling or pushed.

14. What are some other symptoms of Parkinson disease?

Secondary symptoms may be a combination of one or more primary symptoms, or may occur less frequently, or they may be relatively minor. Some secondary symptoms, however, can result in major disability. Not everyone with PD has the same number or mix of secondary symptoms—they vary from person to person. Understanding these symptoms can reduce their impact on your life. Bladder malfunction, constipation, drooling, and walking difficulties are all secondary symptoms of PD that are discussed later.

Loss of smell (Anosmia)

Anosmia may be an early symptom of PD. It results from a loss of dopamine cells in a region of the brain called the **olfactory cortex**. Odors of familiar things such as freshly brewed coffee, baked bread, or perfume may no longer be noticed or appreciated. Loss of smell can also affect one's sense of taste, leading to decreased appetite and weight loss. PD patients who lose their appetite due to anosmia may find they enjoy highly seasoned or spiced foods.

Muscle pain

Pain from dystonia: A muscle cramp or "charley horse" is a strong, painful contraction or tightening of a muscle or group of muscles that comes on suddenly and lasts from a few seconds to several hours. It usually occurs in your calf or foot (but may also involve your arms, trunk, back and neck) while you're resting in bed or exercising. After the cramp disappears the affected muscle or muscles may be sore for several hours. In PD, a common cause of muscle cramps is dystonia: a prolonged twisting or turning of a muscle or group of muscles. Such

Olfactory cortex
Located within the medial temporal lobes the olfactory complex allows us to identify odors.

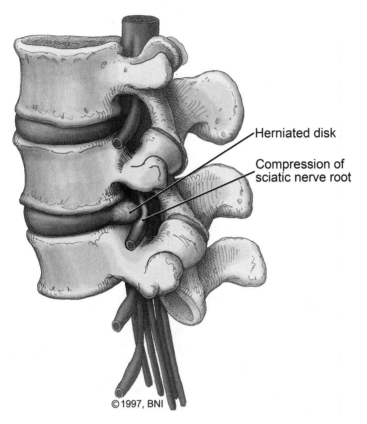

©1997, BNI

Figure 7   Herniated disc.

Figure courtesy of Barrow Neurological Institute.

cramps usually occur at night, when you're resting and medication levels are low. If the pain persists despite adjusting your medications, other causes should be sought. If you are having pain from leg cramps, other causes could be a herniated disc in the back (see **Figure 7**).

Pain from rigidity: A dull gnawing pain like the pain of arthritis or a toothache, affecting your shoulder, neck, back, or hip, your main weight bearing regions, may occur early in PD. Such pain is related to rigidity and disappears when a dopamine agonist such as car-bidopa/levodopa or Stalevo is started.

Treatment of fatigue includes eating a balanced diet and getting adequate rest; exercising regularly but without tiring; improving nighttime sleep; pacing yourself physically, emotionally, and intellectually,

It is important to remember that people with PD can have pain for other reasons, the same ones as people without PD. When pain is severe and persistent, it must not be assumed it is related to PD and other causes should be sought.

Fatigue

More than 50% of people with PD complain of fatigue and, in some, fatigue is one of their most disabling symptoms. Fatigue may mean different things to different people. For some, fatigue refers to drowsiness, for others, it may refer to mental or physical depletion. Some patients may feel a combination of all three.

Treatment of fatigue includes eating a balanced diet and getting adequate rest; exercising regularly but without tiring; improving nighttime sleep; pacing yourself physically, emotionally, and intellectually, because too much stress can aggravate symptoms; adjusting anti-Parkinson drug dosages; and treating depression if applicable.

Facial Masking

Facial masking

A symptom of PD in which the muscles of the face can no longer move, creating an expressionless, mask-like demeanor.

Facial masking, or hypomimia, is a loss of facial expression resulting in a "poker" or "masked face" (as though a person is wearing a mask). The masking results in patients not blinking their eyes, not smiling, and often looking sad. Facial masking is due to rigidity and slowness of the facial muscles and is often one of the first symptoms to improve with anti-Parkinson drugs.

Handwriting

Micrographia is small, cramped handwriting that results from a combination of slowness of movement, incompleteness of movement, and rigidity. Over the years, without your being aware of it, your handwriting may become smaller and more cramped, sometimes becoming completely illegible. Writing a simple sentence once a day, such as "This is a sample of my best handwriting," is an excellent way to track your PD: as your symptoms improve, your handwriting becomes bigger and less cramped.

15. Is an overactive bladder part of PD?

Bladder problems, such as urinary frequency, can be a frustrating and embarrassing effect of PD-related symptoms. The bladder is a smooth muscle, called the **detrusor**, which is shaped like a hollow pyramid with its apex pointed down (see **Figure 8**). The bladder does not contract voluntarily like your arm and leg muscles. Rather it contracts and relaxes in response to how much urine it holds. Normally, your bladder holds approximately 650 ml of urine. As you age, your bladder becomes less elastic and only holds half as much urine.

Detrusor

The bladder is a smooth muscle, called the detrusor.

Contraction of the bladder is regulated by the chemical messengers, norepinephrine and acetylcholine. For your bladder to empty, contraction of the detrusor must be accompanied by relaxation or opening of two sphincters or "locks." The contraction of your internal sphincter is involuntary, while the contraction of your external sphincter is voluntary; this is what allows you to hold your urine until you reach a bathroom. The contraction of both sphincters is under the control of acetylcholine.

If the time and place for urination is appropriate, your conscious brain, your urination center, and your autonomic nervous system (ANS) all work together to contract your bladder and at the same time relax your internal and external sphincters and the voluntary

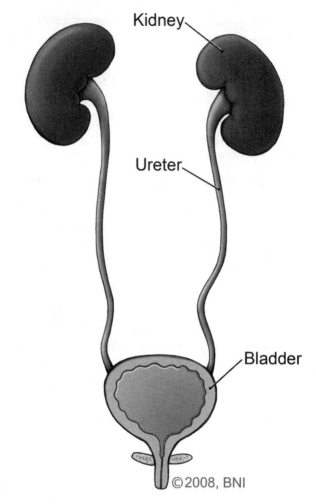

Figure 8   Urinary Tract

Figure courtesy of Barrow Neurological Institute.

muscles of your pelvic floor to allow you to urinate. If your urination center or ANS malfunctions, as either might in PD, you may have symptoms of an overactive bladder, depending on the degree to which the different parts of your nervous system are affected. Less commonly, you might experience symptoms of an underactive (hypoactive or hypotonic) bladder or both an overactive and underactive bladder. In men, an enlarged prostate gland may block the flow of urine. In women, lax pelvic muscles (from child-bearing) may cause incontinence (involuntary loss of urine). The following are the more common symptoms of bladder malfunction in PD:

- *Frequency*, a symptom of an overactive bladder, is a need to void many times, eight or more times a day.
- *Hesitancy*, a symptom of an overactive bladder, is defined as a lag period, several seconds to minutes, between the time you want to void and are at the toilet, but are unable to do so.
- *Incontinence*, an accidental or involuntary loss or leakage of urine. Incontinence may be a symptom of an overactive bladder: you have the urge to void, but can't get to the toilet in time. Or it may be a symptom of a hypotonic bladder, called **overflow incontinence**: urine escaping from a full bladder through a lax sphincter.
- *Stress incontinence* is loss of urine that occurs with coughing, crying, laughing, or sneezing. These activities increase pressure in the abdomen, forcing urine through a lax sphincter.
- *Nocturia*, two or more trips to the bathroom at night is usually a symptom of an overactive bladder or an enlarged prostate or both. At night, when you lie down, your bladder assumes a recumbent position. Instead of concentrating at the bladder-neck, urine spreads out over a larger surface which "fools" your ANS into believing your bladder is fuller than it is. In many people, nocturia causes difficulty sleeping. To minimize nocturia do not drink anything at night and try to avoid alcohol, which is a diuretic. You may also want to try sleeping in an upright position, as this concentrates urine in your bladder neck.

Overflow incontinence

Continual leakage of urine due to the bladder being constantly full.

Hypotonic bladder

In which the bladder fails to empty completely and the urine dribbles out the urethra.

If you have symptoms of an overactive or hypotonic bladder, you should consult a doctor, preferably a urologist.

- *Retention,* an inability to void, is a symptom of an underactive or **hypotonic bladder**. Total inability to void is an emergency and requires catheterization, the insertion of a thin walled tube into the bladder through the urethra.

If you have symptoms of an overactive or hypotonic bladder, you should consult a doctor, preferably a urologist. He or she will give you an examination that includes a urine analysis to rule out an infection. Exams also include blood tests to screen for kidney disease and diabetes. In men, it will include a rectal examination to assess the prostate gland. In women, it will consist of a pelvic examination to assess the bladder, uterus, the relationship of the uterus to the bladder, and firmness of the pelvic muscles.

Treatment for bladder concerns varies depending on the nature of the problem. A urologist can prescribe drugs to relax the bladder and sphincters of an overactive bladder. Acetylcholine blockers such as darifenacin (Enablex), oxybuynin (Ditropan), solifenacin (Vesicare), tolterodine (Detrol), and trospium (Sanctura) work to relax the bladder muscles, but may cause side effects such as dry mouth, blurred vision, constipation, a rapid heartbeat, and flushing, due to blocking the actions of acetylcholine at other sites. In older patients, and some patients with PD, side effects may include confusion, disorientation, delusions, hallucinations, and memory loss. These particular side effects can mimic dementia, but are reversible upon stopping the drugs. However, Enablex and Sanctura do not cross into the brain and do not cause side effects that mimic dementia. Norepinephrine blockers, such as tamsulosin (Flomax), doxazosin (Cardura), terazosin (Hytrin), and alfuzosin (UroXatral) also relax the bladder. Side effects from blocking the actions of norepinephrine at other sites can include low blood pressure, which results in dizziness and fainting.

Kegel exercises (tightening the muscles of the pelvic floor) work to improve urinary and rectal continence and are beneficial to both men and women. The exercises take time to work—it may be 4–8 weeks before you feel the effects. The usual way of identifying the relevant muscles to focus on is to start urinating, then stop mid-stream. The tightening you feel when doing this are the muscles of the pelvic floor. When you restart the flow of urine, you release these pelvic floor muscles. Once identified, you can practice contracting and releasing these muscles independently of urination. One technique to practice is to contract the muscles of your pelvic floor slowly and hold for five seconds, then slowly release. Do this 25 times a day and you will notice a difference.

16. Is constipation part of PD?

Constipation is a common complaint of people with PD. Not having a daily bowel movement isn't constipation, though; **constipation** is defined as two or fewer bowel movements per week. Defecating difficulty is defined as straining at, and incomplete evacuation of, stool. Constipation and defecating difficulty may or may not occur together, and affect up to 50% of PD patients. It is important to distinguish between constipation and defecating difficulty because their treatments differ.

Constipation
Difficulty in passing stool.

Normally, the muscles of your large bowel (colon) propel stool forward. These muscles are controlled by signals from the vagus nerve through part of the ANS, which is affected in PD and sometimes causes the colon's muscles not to fully contract. The passage of stool through the colon then slows, causing the stool to remain in the colon longer, where it hardens and becomes difficult to expel by your rectal muscles. Medications prescribed for PD or other problems may also lead to constipation. For instance, drugs prescribed to regulate your bladder, blood pressure or heart rate all affect the ANS and thus may affect your bowels. PD drugs such as trihexiphenidyl (Artane), benztropine (Cogentin), and amantadine (Symmetrel) block a chemical called acetylcholine, used as a messenger by the vagus nerve, and so these anti-acetylcholine (also called anticholinergic) drugs cause constipation. Similarly, drugs used to treat an overactive bladder (such as Detrol or Ditropan) are also anticholinergics and they too cause constipation. Conversely, drugs used to treat Alzheimer's disease and Lewy body dementia (Aricept, Exelon, Razadyne) increase acetylcholine and may cause diarrhea.

A common cause of constipation in people with and without PD is a diet low in fiber.

A common cause of constipation in people with and without PD is a diet low in fiber. As your colon "transit time" (the time stool stays in your colon) slows, water is absorbed from your stool, making it hard. Fiber, in addition to cleansing your bowel, acts like sawdust, soaking up water, allowing it to remain in your stool and preventing your stool from drying out and becoming hard. Fiber can be *soluble* (dissolves easily) or *insoluble* (passes through the bowel largely unchanged). Americans eat an average of only 5–14 grams of fiber daily, which is short of the 20–35 grams recommended by the American Dietetic Association. Increased dietary fiber is an important first step to avoiding constipation. High-fiber foods include beans, bran, whole grains, and most fresh fruits and vegetables including apples, asparagus, bananas, cabbage, carrots and sprouts. Low fiber foods include cheese, ice cream, milk and most processed foods. Such foods should be avoided if you are constipated. Water and fruit and vegetable juices add fluid to your bowels, bulk-up your stools and make them softer and easier to pass. Drinking at least six 8-ounce glasses of water or fruit/vegetable juice every day can relieve constipation. Caffeinated beverages such as coffee, cola, and tea, and alcoholic beverages, dry and harden your stools, making them more difficult to pass. Constipation is improved by exercise and aggravated by a lack of exercise. Thus, mobile patients are less likely to be constipated than are wheelchair- or bed-bound patients. An hour of exercise per day may do more to lessen constipation than a laxative.

Constipation and the resultant straining can result in several complaints, such as hemorrhoids (dilated and enlarged rectal veins), anal fissures (tears in the skin around the anus), or rectal prolapse (a part of your intestines "popping out" of your rectum). All of these conditions are painful, can bleed, are worrisome, and require prompt medical attention. In a small number of patients (about 5%), a combination of constipation and defecating difficulty results in fecal impaction: an inability to evacuate stool. The pain and discomfort from fecal impaction may be severe and require a visit to the Emergency Department. All of these conditions can be avoided by alleviating constipation. If you have recently become constipated, consult your doctor who may order tests to determine the cause.

In PD, defecating difficulty results from rigidity and/or slowness of contraction of both your abdominal muscles and your gluteal muscles (the muscles with which you sit on the toilet). To expel your stool you must increase the pressure in your abdomen, tightening both your abdominal and gluteal muscles. If you are out of shape, whether you have PD or not, you may be unable to effectively tighten the necessary muscles. Add the rigidity and bradykinesia of PD to your deconditioned muscles and you'll have defecating difficulty despite a proper diet and potent laxatives. Exercising on a daily basis, and thus keeping your abdominal and gluteal muscles in shape, helps a lot.

Patients who are taking levodopa/carbidopa or Stalevo should consider taking their first dose an hour before they are ready for a bowel movement, which will allow the effects of the medication to "kick in" and overcome the rigidity of their abdominal and gluteal muscles. Though rare, in some PD patients the anal sphincter contracts when it should relax. This can be treated by manually relaxing the sphincter, and sometimes by the injection of Botox. If this occurs, avoid excessive straining. If you feel you cannot expel the stool in your rectum, it may help to sit straight up (rather than bend forward), thereby increasing the leverage of your abdominal muscles, allowing them to contract more forcibly. Some patients put a trapeze over their toilet and hold onto it with their hands as they push down with their abdominal muscles, increasing the leverage of those muscles and simultaneously straightening their spine.

The following are additional treatments for constipation and defecating difficulty, arranged in order of their simplicity.

Bran: the outer coating or shell on grain which is removed during processing and found commonly in wheat, oats, and brown rice. One tablespoon of raw bran contains two grams of dietary fiber; start with

1–2 tbsp of bran in a glass daily and gradually increase to three times a day. If you have diverticulitis, ask your doctor if you can use bran. Depending on how long you've been constipated, improvement may take days to weeks.

Psyllium: a naturally occurring dietary fiber made from the ground husks of the psyllium seed. Psyllium holds water and its use results in bulky, easy-to-pass stool. Metamucil is a popular brand of psyllium.

Stool softeners: over-the-counter medications that moisten the stool, making it easier to pass.

Laxatives: some PD patients need a laxative to help expel their stool. Each of the following laxatives works differently; some may work better for you than others. Before using a laxative or a combination of laxatives, speak to your doctor.

- Stimulant laxatives increase the contractions of your colon. Dulcolax and Senokot are brand names for this type of laxative. Dulcolax can be taken as a pill or administered as a suppository.
- Mineral or osmotic laxatives act like "sponges," drawing water into the colon, making it easier to pass stool. Milk of Magnesia, Miralax, and Lactulose are popular over-the-counter brands, all of which should have an effect within 12 to 24 hours. These laxatives should be used only with your doctor's knowledge and not for more than two weeks at a time. Over-usage may result in nausea, diarrhea, and possibly, electrolyte imbalances (excessive loss of sodium and/or potassium in the stool). Amitiza (lubiprostone) is a prescription drug that increases the secretion of water into the bowel via the chloride channel, allowing the stool to pass more easily.

17. Is drooling part of PD?

Drooling

The discharge of saliva from the mouth.

Drooling (sialorrhea), or excessive saliva, results from difficulty swallowing and is a frequent symptom in PD. Most of the time, drooling is merely an annoyance. However, sometimes it's an embarrassment, and sometimes it's even a hazard: aspiration of saliva (swallowing saliva into your lungs) can cause pneumonia.

Saliva is the watery liquid that coats your food, making it slippery and easier to swallow. Saliva contains enzymes that break down complex carbohydrates and starches, making them easier to digest, and also contains bactericidal chemicals that fight tooth decay. Swallowing removes saliva and prevents it from accumulating in your mouth and throat. It is an active process requiring coordination of the circular muscles of your throat and esophagus. In PD, the muscles of your tongue, palate, throat, and esophagus may be affected, becoming rigid and slow and losing their ability to propel food downward. Gravity also aids in swallowing. During the day, when your head is erect (when you are seated or standing), saliva is propelled by your tongue, palate, and throat, and moves down your esophagus into your stomach. At night, however, with your head down, gravity no longer helps and saliva drips onto your pillow. You may wake in the morning to a wet pillow.

Saliva is produced by your salivary glands: the parotid, sub-maxillary, and sub-lingual glands located in the floor of your mouth and at the angle of the jaw. Although the production of saliva is automatic, production can be increased in response to eternal events, such as the sight, smell, or taste of food (even the thought of food). The ANS controls the production of saliva through releasing acetylcholine, which stimulates receptors on cells of the salivary glands. In addition to the rigidity of your throat and esophageal muscles associated with PD, drooling may also result from increased production of saliva secondary to over-activity of your ANS.

The first approach to treating drooling is education. Understanding the reasons you drool can help you tackle the cause. For example, sleeping with your head raised allows gravity to help you swallow your saliva. Chewing sugarless gum stimulates the circular muscles of your throat and also helps you swallow your saliva. These suggestions help, but eventually, as PD progresses, they may not be enough. The next approach is use of anticholinergic drugs, which block the actions of acetylcholine at **cholinergic receptors** on the salivary glands. Artane and Cogentin both work in this way to decrease drooling. Trihexiphenidyl also blocks acetylcholine receptors in your body, but may cause confusion, delusions, memory loss, blurred vision, constipation, and/or urinary retention. Few patients can tolerate the high doses required to control drooling without side effects. Darifenacin (Enablex) and trospium (Sanctura) are anticholinergic drugs that are helpful in treating overactive bladder. As neither drug enters the brain, both can be used to treat drooling without causing confusion, delusions, or memory loss. However, these drugs are expensive and as they are not yet FDA-approved to control drooling, it is unlikely your insurance company will pay for them. For some people, however, the price is worth the result.

One final approach is **Botox** (botulinum toxin), which is a large protein molecule that blocks the release of acetylcholine onto muscles and can stop the secretion of acetylcholine by the salivary glands. Because of its size, it is difficult for Botox to go anywhere and thus

Tell Me More

Chewing sugarless gum stimulates the circular muscles of your throat and also helps you swallow your saliva.

Cholinergic receptors

Enzymes in cells that attach to acetylcholine.

Botox

A large protein molecule that blocks the release of acetylcholine onto muscles and can stop the secretion of acetylcholine by the salivary glands.

the effects are confined to the site of injection. When injecting Botox for drooling, care must be taken to avoid the muscles of swallowing located at the base of the mouth. Such an injection can temporarily cause an inability to swallow.

18. Is a stooped posture part of PD?

In observing and treating 50 PD patients and their 46 spouses, the most important observation this author made was that 90% of the patients, all of whom maintained their ability to walk 20 to 40 years post-PD diagnosis, had a straight spine. These patients and their elderly spouses did not stoop, paid attention to keeping their spine straight, and exercised at least an hour a day, continuing to keep their spine straight while doing so.

The spine is a lever to which the muscles that flex and extend your hips are attached. They're among the most powerful muscles of your legs, the muscles that propel you forward. If your spine is straight, your hip flexors and extensors work optimally. If your spine is bent and you look toward the floor, it is difficult to walk with more than short shuffling steps—like someone with PD. Walking this way, you are more likely to fatigue easily and to fall. In PD, for reasons yet unknown, the spine begins to bend. It could simply be an adjustment by your body to maintain a center of gravity. Or it could be **dystonia**—an unequal pull of the muscles that flex or bend the spine; **atrophy**—a weakening of the muscles that extend or straighten your spine; or osteoporosis. It is estimated that 50% of women and 25% of men with PD have osteoporosis. A bent spine is more likely to lead to falls, swelling of the legs, and blood clots forming in the veins of your legs (a condition known as phlebitis).

Dystonia

Involuntary muscle spasms resulting in awkward and sustained postures, which may be painful. Dystonia can involve the eyes, neck, the trunk, and the limbs.

Atrophy

A weakening of the muscles that extend or straighten your spine.

A bent spine leads to your neck bending forward, making it more difficult to both chew and swallow your food. It also creates difficulty speaking loudly and clearly. To speak or sing loudly and clearly, one's spine must be straight and chin held up. The muscles of speaking and swallowing overlap; they both require the leverage of a straight spine in order to work effectively.

Many people with PD complain of shortness of breath, though their hearts and lungs may check out as normal in an exam, because the problem is with the intercostal muscles—muscles between your ribs—which are your respiratory muscles. These muscles are affected by both aging and PD; for them to work best, your spine must be straight, giving them maximum leverage. Your diaphragm (an accessory muscle of respiration) also works best when you are upright and your spine is straight. Sit quietly, breath normally, and count how many breaths you take in one minute. If you are taking more than 20 breaths per minute, you are likely not using the muscles of your chest wall optimally. Keeping your spine straight may help you breathe better.

As your spine bends, your muscles don't work as effectively; they no longer massage your veins effectively and this can cause fluid to back up into your feet and legs. This swelling, or edema, can have other causes, such as heart failure, pelvic obstruction, high sodium diet, or reaction to medication. However, in many older people and those with PD, the swelling is related to inefficiency of the leg muscles. A bent spine causes the leg muscles to work at a mechanical disadvantage; they do not pump as hard or as well and cannot propel fluid from the feet to the heart, causing that fluid to accumulate in the feet. Raising your feet above your heart or massaging your legs will help the fluid "drain" back to the heart, but the best method is to start exercises that will help you maintain a straight spine and build stronger leg muscles.

Many older people and people with PD have difficulty maintaining their balance. They walk well, but can easily fall.

Many older people and people with PD have difficulty maintaining their balance. They walk well, but can easily fall. When they fall they are unable to react quickly enough to catch themselves and break their fall. When you trip, information about the changing position of your body in space is subconsciously relayed to your brain through sensors in your feet, inner ears, and your eyes. Your body will take corrective actions to prevent or break your fall before you even realize you are falling. These corrective actions are called "righting reflexes:" reflexes that right, or correct, your position in space. Unfortunately, a bent spine impairs your righting reflexes. The exercises described in this book may improve your balance and your righting reflexes by helping you to maintain a straight spine.

Because your spine bends without your being aware of it, it is difficult to correct. Your brain is meant to survey the outside world and alert you to danger, not to keep track of your spine. Such "ordinary" housekeeping chores are assigned to a part of your subconscious brain called the basal ganglia. The basal ganglia, when they are not affected by age or PD, maintain the correct tone of the flexor and extensor muscles of your spine. When, however, they are affected by age and PD, the flexor muscles pull more than the extensor muscles, and your spine flexes or bends.

The pull of the flexor muscles on your spine is constant: when you are sitting, standing, and walking. Exercises to strengthen the opposing muscles help, but alone will not reverse the bending. To counteract the downward pull on the muscles of your spine, you must adapt strategies or habits that minimize it. I recommend the following:

The Buddha habit. Sit on a chair with your legs wide apart, approximating the Buddha's "lotus position." This forces your hip joints out, raises your pelvis, and straightens out your spine. Each time you sit, sit with your legs wide apart and lean your elbows on an arm-rest; this elevates your shoulder blades and further straightens out your spine. If you are sitting in a chair without arm-rests, raise your elbows and press your palms together—this also will straighten your spine.

The John F. Kennedy rocking chair. President John F. Kennedy had a bad back and used a rocking chair to relieve his pain. A rocking chair is an excellent way to maintain a straight spine, to relieve the pressure of a "bad" back, and to exercise the muscles of your legs. Choose a rocker that you can straddle, one foot on the outside of each rocker—this raises your pelvis and straightens out your spine. Lean your elbows on the arm rest—this raises your shoulder blades and further straightens your spine. Now rock! It's a great exercise for the flexors and extensors of your hips, knees, and feet.

The General Patton stance. Stand with your hands on your hips—like General George Patton. This auto-matically forces your shoulder blades up and straight-ens out your spine. If your spine is straight you are exerting maximum leverage on the muscles of your legs; your balance will be better, you will be less likely to fall and less likely to tire. A variant on standing with your hands on your hips is to stand with your arms behind your back, hands entwined. This posture is called "parade rest."

Think "Surprise!" While seated, raise your hands above your head, as though you are saying, "surprise." Keep your elbows straight, reach back, and slowly touch the wall with the back of your hands. You'll feel a pull on the extensor muscles of your spine and neck, a tug that counteracts the downward pull on them. Do this exercise 20 times a day; it supplements the habits you've learned to straighten your spine.

Breathing. Your ribs are attached to your spine at a 90 degree angle. If your spine is bent, your intercostal muscles are forced into an acute angle, creating a mechanical disadvantage, and they do not work as efficiently. If your spine is straight, the full effect of gravity is exerted on your diaphragm. Your diaphragm makes fuller, more complete excursions, and thus you breathe more efficiently. A bent spine limits the movement of your diaphragm, causing you to breathe faster and shallower, spend more energy on the mechanics of breathing, and become short of breath. If your intercostal muscles and your diaphragm are not working efficiently, you are less able to cough and to bring up the secretions and food particles that can lodge in your lungs, which can lead to pneumonia.

Chewing and swallowing. If your spine is straight, your neck is also straight, and you can chew and swallow better. Chewing with an extended neck allows you to grind your food easily, with less likelihood of having a large particle of food get stuck in your throat. When your spine is straight and your chin is up, your muscles of mastication (those you use for chewing) have a mechanical advantage and thus chewing is easier.

Swallowing, however, is more complex than chewing. To swallow, you must flex your neck to prevent food from lodging in your windpipe. If there is something wrong with your teeth, gums, or throat, you will have difficulty swallowing and you will be fully aware of it. If, however, the trouble swallowing arises because of age, or disease of the basal ganglia, you may not initially be aware of the trouble. The first clue may be an unexplained weight loss, or coughing or choking while eating. The coughing and choking are attempts by your body to get rid of the food that is sticking in your throat or getting into your lungs. If you are having difficulty chewing your food, try straddling your chair. This forces your spine, neck, and chin up. Then sit with your elbows on the table, further forcing your spine, neck, and chin up. If you make it a habit to sit while straddling your chair and keeping your elbows on the table, you will chew and swallow better, and you will be less likely to aspirate (get food caught in your throat).

19. Is difficulty speaking part of PD?

About half of all PD patients have difficulty speaking. The difficulty ranges in severity from minor to moderate in most patients, and marked in about 10%. Minor difficulties may be barely perceptible to most listeners and not at all perceptible to the patient. Minor difficulties in speaking are best appreciated over the telephone: the phone filters out many high frequencies and makes your speech less audible. Marked difficulties are usually associated with difficulty in swallowing and breathing. The muscles used in speaking are shared, in part, by the muscles used in swallowing and breathing, and when one set is severely affected it is likely the other sets will also be affected.

Speech can be divided into voice, the act and the mechanics of speaking, and language, the content of

About half of all PD patients have difficulty speaking. The difficulty ranges in severity from minor to moderate

speech. PD mainly affects voice. Strokes of the left-side of the brain, PD dementia (Lewy body dementia), and Alzheimer's disease, all affect language. The qualities of voice affected by PD are: loudness, tone (the vocal "equivalent" of the shades of a particular color, like the different shades of blue or red or yellow), and pitch (the vocal equivalent of the intensity, the brightness or darkness, of a particular shade of color). For most PD patients, voice difficulty manifests as a *decrease* in loudness, tone, and pitch. Your voice may be described as low, monotonous, and unvarying. Voice difficulty in PD, like difficulty moving, arises because the muscles involved in speaking are affected: they become rigid, they move slowly and incompletely. These muscles and the structures they affect include the nose, lips, tongue, cheeks, soft and hard palates, back of the throat or pharynx, vocal cords, and the muscles of the chest wall including the diaphragm and the intercostal muscles.

Your vocal cords are muscles; their configuration results from an in-folding of a membrane stretched across the larynx, or voice box. The cords vibrate, modulating the flow of air coming from your lungs.

Your vocal cords are muscles; their configuration results from an in-folding of a membrane stretched across the larynx, or voice box. The cords vibrate, modulating the flow of air coming from your lungs. The frequency at which your cords vibrate determines the pitch of your voice; females have a higher frequency than males, and thus higher-pitched voices. Three problems related to the vocal cords can occur in PD:

First, your cords may not close completely. This can be seen by examining the cords through an instrument called a laryngoscope. If your cords don't close completely, your voice becomes low and muffled. In some patients, collagen may be injected into each cord to "bulk it up," resulting in more complete closure.

Second, your vocal cords may close too tightly. This can also be seen through a laryngoscope. If your cords close too tightly, your voice, while initially loud, fades quickly, and has a "reedy" or "breathy" quality. In some patients the cords close too tightly because of scarring, and in some because of dystonia, called spasmodic dystonia, which can be helped by Botox injections into the vocal cords. In Parkinson-like conditions such as multiple system atrophy, the cords may close completely. Such closure is heralded by a shrill, high-pitched sound called strider. This is a medical emergency because, if not treated, air will be unable to enter your lungs from your nose and throat.

Third, and most common, the vocal cords may not vibrate as rapidly and may fatigue easily. This is responsible, in part, for the low, monotonous voice common in PD patients.

Your lungs also play a role in the quality of your voice. Housed in your chest wall cavity, your lungs are protected by the bony structure of your rib cage and further enclosed by a double-walled sac called the pleura. Your intercostal muscles work to expand and contract your chest cavity as you breathe, allowing air into your lungs through your trachea and bronchial tubes. In PD, your intercostal muscles become rigid, which can result in your breathing faster—up to 20 breaths or more per minute. This faster rate of breathing, called hyperventilation, results in a decrease in the carbon dioxide tension and in the buffering capacity of your blood, leading to a feeling of shortness of breath or suffocation, which fatigues you and heightens anxiety.

If you are unable to take a deep breath, you cannot speak loudly. To illustrate this, hold your breath and

First, place a helium-quality balloon between your lips, tightening and toning the lip muscles. Slowly blow up the balloon, tightening and toning your cheek, throat, and intercostal muscles. Do this 30 times a day when your anti-Parkinson drugs are working and your muscles are working efficiently.

Lee Silverman Voice Therapy

A method of training a person to strengthen his or her voice by singing loudly or shouting.

American Academy of Neurology

It is a professional society for neurologists and neuroscientists.

try to speak loudly. Your voice, initially loud, quickly fades. As disorders of the vocal cords are difficult to treat, I emphasize improving the other muscles involved in speaking. The regimen I teach is one that can be easily carried out by anyone, anywhere. First, place a helium-quality balloon between your lips, tightening and toning the lip muscles. Slowly blow up the balloon, tightening and toning your cheek, throat, and intercostal muscles. Do this 30 times a day when your anti-Parkinson drugs are working and your muscles are working efficiently.

Therapists who treat PD are usually familiar with or trained in the **Lee Silverman Voice Therapy** (LSVT). LSVT emphasized voice training by strengthening the muscles used in speaking; similar to training an opera singer to sing louder. At the Muhammad Ali Parkinson Center (MAPC), patients are taught to speak louder and more clearly.

20. I am seeing a neurologist—what should I expect?

Although your primary care doctor may have recognized the symptoms of PD, he or she is trained primarily in family medicine or internal medicine and may see few people with PD. Although primary care doctors recognize the symptoms of PD, they may not be up-to-date on all the latest developments and treatments, nor have they had the neurological training to deal effectively with it.

To confirm a diagnosis of PD it is best to see a neurologist—better yet, a neurologist who specializes in PD, called a movement disorder specialist. To find a neurologist nearby, contact the **American Academy of Neurology** (www.aan.com), which maintains a list of neurologists. Likewise, the **Movement Disorder Society** (www.movementdisorders.org) maintains a list of movement disorder specialists. Because treating PD requires more than an occasional visit, it is important to find a neurologist with whom you can have a good working relationship. Like any chronic disease, it requires that you and your family work together with the neurologist to find the best treatment or treatments. A knowledgeable neurologist can provide more than medicine to treat your symptoms: he or she can provide understanding, advice, and reassurance.

At your first visit, the neurologist will want to know why you came, your medical history, your family history (especially a history of PD or tremor), and what, if anything, in your history may have contributed to your symptoms. Bring a summary of your medical history, including serious and chronic illnesses, hospitalizations, surgeries, allergies, drugs taken, and lifestyle risks. If what you have to talk about feels difficult, or if you're likely to forget what's said, bring a trusted friend or family member with you.

The doctor or his assistant may ask about your **activities of daily living** (**ADLs**) (see **Table 3**), which will likely include questions about speech, salivation, swallowing, handwriting, cutting food and handling utensils, dressing, hygiene, turning in bed, falling, freezing, walking, tremor, and sensory symptoms. Any and all of these areas may be affected by PD and the neurologist's careful questioning may help determine how the disease is progressing.

The neurological examination covers several areas. Rigidity is examined by testing muscle tone at your wrists, elbows, shoulders, and knees by holding the limb

Tell Me More

Movement disorder

Any of a number of conditions that affect a person's ability to move normally, or that cause abnormal, involuntary movements.

To confirm a diagnosis of PD it is best to see a neurologist— better yet, a neurologist who specializes in PD, called a movement disorder specialist.

Activities of daily living (ADLs)

Activities usually performed for oneself in the course of a normal day including bathing, dressing, grooming, eating, walking, using the telephone, taking medications, and other personal care activities.

Table 3   Activities of Daily Living

	0	1	2	3	4
Speech	Normal	Mildly affected	Moderately affected	Severely affected	Can't speak
Salivation	Normal	Slight drooling	Moderate drooling	Marked drooling	Severe drooling
Swallowing	Normal	Rare choking	Frequent choking	Needs soft food	Has feeding tube
Handwriting	Normal	Slightly small	Moderately small	Mostly illegible	Entirely illegible
Feeding	Normal	Slow, no help	Some help	Much help	Can't feed self
Dressing	Normal	Slow, no help	Some help	Much help	Can't dress self
Hygiene	Normal	Slow, no help	Some help	Much help	Can't do
Tremor	None	Slight	Moderate	Severe	Very severe
Falls	None	Rare	Some	Fall 1/day	Falls more than 1/day
Freezes when walking	None	Rare	Occasional fall or freeze	Frequent freeze; occasional fall	Frequent fall or freeze
Walking	Normal	Drags leg	Short steps, no help	Needs cane or walker	Can't walk
Turning in bed	Normal	Slow, no help	Some help	Much help	Can't turn
Ache, cramp, pain in legs	None	Occasional ache; hurt in leg	Frequent ache; hurt in legs	Frequent pain, leg cramps	Severe pain, leg cramps

and moving it both slowly and rapidly. The testing of **deep tendon reflexes,** by tapping with a rubber reflex hammer on the tendons at your jaw, elbows, knees, and ankles, reveals much to an examiner. The examiner will note if the reflexes are increased on one side of your body versus the other (as after a stroke), whether they are increased in your legs versus your arms (as in a myelopathy—see below), or if they are absent (as in damage to the nerves in your arms and legs). In PD the deep tendon reflexes are normal, but in some of the Parkinson-like disorders they may be increased.

Testing of strength or power provides insight into how your nervous system works. Rapid alternating movements of your hands and feet are tested by asking you to tap your fingers to your thumb, turn the palms of your hands up and down, turn your wrists from side to side as though you're screwing in a light bulb, and move your feet up and down as though you're walking. The examiner will observe the speed, amplitude and rhythm of your movements and compare your left with your right side. Rapid alternating movements are decreased in PD.

Tests of coordination are carried out by asking you to touch your finger to your nose and then to the tip of the neurologist's finger. Another test involves running the heel of one foot down the shin of the opposite leg. This provides information on a region of your brain called the cerebellum. Coordination is normal in PD, but it may be impaired in some of the Parkinson-like disorders. Eye movements are also evaluated. They are normal in PD, but are impaired in a Parkinson-like disorder called **progressive supranuclear palsy** (PSP).

Speech (the mechanics) is also affected in PD. The neurologist may ask you to say specific words to determine

Deep tendon reflex tests

One of the functions of medical evaluation, conducted by tapping with a rubber reflex hammer on the tendons at your jaw, elbows, knees, and ankles.

Tell Me More

Progressive supranuclear palsy

A movement disorder with symptoms similar to PD.

which muscles are affected. For example, saying the words "mama" or "papa" uses the **orbicularis oris** muscle—your lips. Saying the word "lulu" uses your tongue muscle, while the vowels, "A", "E", "I", "O", "U", are sounds you make with the muscles of your throat.

Orbicularis oris
The lips.

The sensory examination includes an evaluation of your ability to perceive a light touch, such as a pin prick, and your ability to tell (with your eyes closed) whether your thumb or great toe is being moved up or down. Not every neurologist does the same examination; some neurologists may emphasize one part of the examination over another. At the Muhammad Ali Parkinson Center, as in most movement disorder centers, the neurologist will examine you using the motor portion of the Unified Parkinson's Disease Rating Scale (UPDRS). This portion evaluates symptoms such as speech, facial expression, tremor, rigidity, bradykinesia, arising from a chair, posture, turning, walking, and postural stability using the following scale:

0 = normal

1 = minimally impaired

2 = moderately impaired

3 = markedly impaired

4 = unable to perform

An overall score of "0" means there is no disability and "108" indicates complete disability. As in golf, the lower the score, the better you are. As a rule, overall scores of 20 or below indicate relatively mild to moderate disability, while overall scores of 40 or more indicate marked disability. Sometimes a neurologist will evaluate you in the morning after you have gone 12 to

24 hours without carbidopa/levodopa, then again one hour after a test dose of carbidopa/levodopa. This often provides you and the neurologist with insight into the state of the underlying disease and its responsiveness to anti-Parkinson drugs.

21. How can I make my visit to a neurologist successful?

Your visit to the neurologist is successful if, upon leaving the office, you know what's wrong and what the neurologist can do to make you better. The visit is less successful if, upon leaving the office, you don't know what's wrong, but the neurologist has told you, in words you can understand, why he or she doesn't know what's wrong—and can tell you what he or she will do to find out what's wrong. An unsuccessful visit is one in which you leave the office without knowing what's wrong and the neurologist can't tell you how he or she will determine the problem. Ideally you should not leave the neurologist's office feeling more anxious, depressed, and confused than before. Even in this age of shorter visits, harried doctors, and more complicated problems, there are steps you can take to make your visit as successful as possible. Start by asking yourself why you're seeing the neurologist. If you can't explain "why" in a few words, the neurologist might not be able to help. He or she is a neurologist, not a mind reader, and needs to hear from you what the problem is before trying to address it.

When you visit the neurologist, you may be anxious or depressed, thinking: "What's wrong? Is it bad? Will the neurologist know—and be able to help?" You may be angry (whether you realize it or not), thinking: "Why me? Why do I have to have a disease of the brain? Why

Your visit to the neurologist is successful if, upon leaving the office, you know what's wrong and what the neurologist can do to make you better.

do I have to see a neurologist? And why do I have to pay for the privilege?" While they are perfectly understandable, try not to let these thoughts overwhelm you or get in your way of understanding this disease. If, after being diagnosed, you don't agree with or like the diagnosis, don't "shoot the messenger." The neurologist may be wrong, in which case you're likely to resent the message all the more, but the neurologist may be right—and resenting the messenger doesn't change the message! Remember, you are the one who might have PD and needs help; the neurologist is there to help you.

If you think you have PD, or your family doctor thinks you have PD and refers you to a specialist, you may wonder how to determine if the specialist is good. If your family doctor picked the specialist, it probably means that your doctor has worked with him or her before, and knows the specialist's credentials and abilities. However, in an era where Health Maintenance Organizations (HMOs) and insurance companies limit some choices, this may not be the case. Ask your family doctor, or the specialist (or the specialist's office manager) the following questions:

1. *Is the specialist a neurologist?* To practice as a neurologist a doctor, an MD (medical doctor) or a DO (a doctor of osteopathy), must complete an accredited 3-year neurology training program.

2. *Is the neurologist board certified?* Upon completion of their training program, a neurologist takes an examination in neurology and psychiatry. For a neurologist, 75% of the questions are on neurology and 25% are on psychiatry. Upon successful completion of the examination, neurologists are designated by the American Board of Psychiatry and Neurology as being certified in Neurology. Board certification

(as evidenced by a diploma) is like a Good Housekeeping Seal of Approval (although it is not a guarantee of competence). There are exceptions, though; the best neurologist I knew was not board-certified because he wouldn't take the time to bother with the test.

3. *Is the neurologist a movement disorder specialist?* Within the field of neurology, there are accredited (by separate Boards) sub-specialties. Movement disorders (which includes PD) is a sub-specialty, but is not accredited by a separate Board. Movement disorders include PD (approximately 80% of the practice), the PD-like disorders (multiple system atrophy, progressive supranuclear palsy, corticobasilar degeneration, dystonia, essential tremor, Huntington disease, restless leg syndrome, tardive dyskinesia, and Wilson disease). To be called a movement disorder specialist, a neurologist must take a 1- to 3-year fellowship in a movement disorder program after finishing neurology training. Usually, the specialist will display a certificate attesting to completion of the fellowship. If you do not see such a certificate, ask where the specialist trained in movement disorders. There are excellent neurologists who treat PD but did not complete movement disorder fellowships. They may, like most movement disorder specialists, belong to the Movement Disorder Society (MDS). The MDS is an excellent organization, but membership does not guarantee competence; any neurologist or researcher can belong if they pay the annual fee.

Once you have found a neurologist to try, prepare for your first visit. You may be anxious or afraid and be worried that you will not remember everything you want to ask, yet try not to come with a long list. List the 3 or 4 main problems, complaints, or concerns in their order of importance to you. If you're satisfied the

List the 3 or 4 main problems, complaints, or concerns in their order of importance to you. If you're satisfied the doctor has answered your main questions and there are others you want the doctor (and not his staff) to answer, make a return appointment.

doctor has answered your main questions and there are others you want the doctor (and not his staff) to answer, make a return appointment.

If you are seeing the neurologist because you think you have PD, say exactly what prompted you to come. The following are examples: "I think I have PD because I have a tremor." "My wife (or a friend or another doctor) thinks I might have PD." "I saw Muhammad Ali or Michael J. Fox on television and I think I have what they have." If you can, take a family member or friend with you on your first visit to provide emotional support and comfort. They are more likely to be objective and hear what the specialist said, rather than what you thought he said, and can help you to remember what is recommended if you become too overwhelmed or anxious to remember it all. A word of caution: too many family members or friends in the room change the dynamics of the visit. If you have small children, get a babysitter. Children may be frightened by being in a doctor's office, and they can cry and be disruptive.

Look for a courteous, caring, and polite staff, a clean office, and information on PD: books, pamphlets, and newsletters. Look for a nurse or an assistant to ask you to fill out forms containing questions about PD. Such questions tell the neurologist what he or she thinks is important. The questions asked, the clarity with which they are asked, and the detail into which they go will give you an idea as to how the neurologist thinks. Waits of more than half an hour are rarely justified. Before your visit, ask whether the neurologist goes to the hospital before seeing patients. If he or she does, this may result in delays because of unforeseen emergencies. If the neurologist goes to the hospital, ask for an appointment on a day he or she does not go. If you asked the neurologist to "squeeze you in," and he or she did so, expect a delay. A doctor who will see you as an emergency or as a favor will generally set a time he can see you, or he will say, "I cannot fit you in, but I can have my associate or my colleague do so."

Although the diagnosis of PD may be apparent as soon as you walk in, the neurologist should stifle the urge to make a quick diagnosis. To begin with, the diagnosis may be incorrect, or if correct, such a quick diagnosis can be disturbing and not appreciated by you or your family. At the beginning of the disease, you and your family are probably frightened and anxious. You've sensed something's wrong but may have denied or dismissed the symptoms. If a stranger, a neurologist, quickly points out the obvious, it will likely reinforce any guilt you may feel about not seeking help sooner. A recurrent theme of patients seeking another opinion is that the other neurologist "didn't examine me or listen to me." The neurologist must convey a caring attitude; this will help establish a trusting doctor-patient relationship.

After taking a history and doing an examination, the neurologist may order a magnetic resonance imaging (MRI) scan of your brain. An MRI-scan does not confirm or negate the diagnosis of PD, rather it eliminates, or "rules out," other disorders that can mimic PD. For example, an MRI scan of your brain may reveal that your difficulty walking is from a disorder called normal pressure hydrocephalus (NPH) or from multiple small strokes (Vascular Parkinson).

A neurologist may also choose to do a "levodopa test," which involves putting you on a dose of carbidopa/levodopa 3-4 times a day for 4-6 weeks. Patients with PD respond to levodopa, while patients with PD-like disorders respond poorly or not at all. However, I don't do a levodopa test on patients because Parkinson disease can usually be diagnosed without it and once you are started on levodopa it is hard to stop—and there are advantages to delaying levodopa.

22. Is Parkinson disease the reason I have trouble walking?

There are several gait disorders that either may be mistaken for PD or may co-exist with PD. Parkinson disease does not protect you from having another gait disorder. Different gait disorders have different symptoms that help in distinguishing one disorder from another (e.g., whether you take short steps or shuffle while walking, whether you swing your arms while walking, or how easily you fall if pushed backwards, the presence or absence of certain reflexes, the response to levodopa, and the results of an MRI scan of the brain).

Myeolopathy refers to a gait disorder that results from pressure on the upper or cervical spinal cord. It is characterized by a scissor-like gait: your feet turning in like the blades of a scissor when you walk along a straight pathway or when you turn. Examination usually reveals weakness of the legs, the deep tendon reflexes are exaggerated, and your big toes curl up after the doctor scratches the soles of your feet with a pin. This last test is called the Babinski response, after the neurologist who first described it.

Normal Pressure Hydrocephalus. Hydrocephalus is a disorder in which there is too much cerebrospinal fluid in the ventricles of your brain. These ventricles enlarge to accommodate the extra fluid and then press on the brain, causing impairment. Normal pressure hydrocephalus (NPH) is a type of hydrocephalus that occurs

Myleopathy

A gait disorder that results from pressure on the upper or cervical spinal cord.

Normal Pressure Hydrocephalus

Normal pressure hydrocephalus (NPH) is a rise in cerebrospinal fluid (CSF) in the brain that affects brain function.

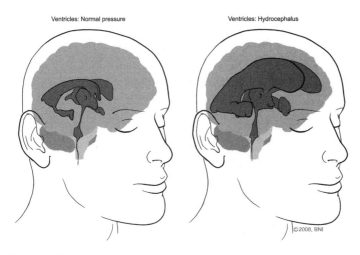

Ventricles: Normal pressure

Ventricles: Hydrocephalus

©2008, BNI

Figure 9   Normal Pressure Hydrocephalus

Figure courtesy of Barrow Neurological Institute.

in older adults, generally 60 years and over. NPH develops gradually, usually over several years. Its exact cause is unknown, although the symptoms are due to the enlarged ventricles pressing on the brain (see **Figure 9**). Symptoms can be grouped into mental symptoms, difficulty walking, and difficulty urinating.

The mental symptoms of NPH can mimic those of Alzheimer's disease (AD) or PD dementia (Lewy body disease): apathy, anxiety, depression, difficulty paying attention, remembering, and thinking. Testing by an experienced neuropsychologist may help in distinguishing among the mental symptoms of AD, PD, and NPH. The gait disorder of NPH can mimic PD, including the short steps, shuffling, unsteadiness, and freezing of gait (FOG) that occurs. The urinary symptoms can either mimic those of PD or of an enlarged prostate gland: frequency, urgency, and incontinence. An experienced neurologist or a movement disorder specialist may, on the basis of his or her examination, suspect NPH.

The mental symptoms of NPH can mimic those of Alzheimer's disease (AD) or PD dementia (Lewy body disease): apathy, anxiety, depression, difficulty paying attention, remembering, and thinking.

Tell Me More

Diagnosis of NPH may begin with an MRI that reveals enlarged ventricles. However, the MRI does not indicate whether the ventricles are enlarged due to hydrocephalus, normal age-related brain atrophy, or the atrophy caused by AD or PD dementia. By comparing the degree of atrophy over the surface of the brain and the size of the ventricles, an experienced neurologist can usually distinguish NPH from brain atrophy. A neuro-radiologist may suggest additional diagnostic tests which vary from center to center. Diagnosis of NPH is also helped by a lumbar puncture (a spinal tap) to measure spinal fluid pressure. An elevated pressure suggests hydro-cephalus rather than brain atrophy. However, NPH can exist in the presence of normal pressure (hence the name normal pressure hydrocephalus). A large amount of **CSF** is removed and analyzed for cells, protein, and sugar. In NPH, the analysis will be negative. The large volume of CSF removed may result in a temporary improvement (24 to 48 hours) of walking difficulty. If such an improvement occurs, it is suggestive of NPH.

Senile Gait/Vascular Parkinson. Shrinkage or atrophy of the brain with a loss of the neurons that regulate walking (senile gait), or a series of strokes that damage the same regions of the brain (vascular PD) can result in a gait disorder that resembles PD. Depending on the degree of atrophy or the location and number of strokes, the walking difficulty of senile gait or vascular PD may include short steps, freezing of gait, and unsteadiness (postural instability). Senile gait may or may not be a forerunner of Alzheimer disease. An experienced neurologist or a movement disorder specialist can usually distinguish senile gait or vascular PD from PD. Examination will include leg muscle tone and how their resistance to being stretched differs. Parkinson disease is

CSF

A watery fluid, continuously produced and absorbed, which flows in the ventricles (cavities) within the brain and around the surface of the brain and spinal cord.

Senile Gait

Shrinkage or atrophy of the brain with a loss of the neurons that regulate walking.

Vascular Parkinson

Condition caused by a cumulative effect of multiple "silent" or "minor" strokes affecting the striatum, globus pallidus, thalamus, cerebellum, and midbrain that cause symptoms similar to PD.

characterized by rigidity, while senile gait and vascular PD by spasticity and gengenhalten (involuntary resistance to passive movement of the extremities). Deep tendon reflexes may be increased in senile gait and vascular PD, but are normal in PD. Babinski signs and a reflex called the "tonic foot" or "grasp" (the sole of the foot gripping the ground) are present in both senile gait and vascular PD, but absent in PD. While walking and leg tone are affected in senile gait and vascular PD, the arms remain unaffected, unlike in PD. Thus in senile gait or vascular PD the arms swing while walking, but one or both don't in PD.

23. What is dystonia?

Dystonia is increased muscle tone, but it results from a different alteration in the nervous system than rigidity or spasticity. Dystonia usually results in your neck, arm, leg, or trunk becoming twisted or turned. An **electromyogram** (EMG), an electrical recording of the muscle firing, usually reveals a distinct pattern, one entirely different from rigidity or spasticity. Dystonia may be a symptom of PD or of one of the PD-like disorders. The cramps that PD patients experience when levodopa is wearing off or when they awaken in the morning are usually leg dystonias.

Electromyogram (EMG)

An electrical recording of the muscle firing.

Acute dystonia, consisting of sustained, sometimes painful muscle spasms that result in abnormal twisting or turning, usually of the head and neck, but sometimes of an arm or a leg, the whole body (ophistotonus), or the eyes (oculogyric crisis), may occur within hours of injecting a neuroleptic (a drug used to treat behavioral disorders such as psychosis or schizophrenia). The acute dystonia may last several hours and is relieved by injecting Benadryl, an antihistamine. About 3–10% of patients treated with a neuroleptic may have an acute dystonia. The risk is higher with drugs such as Haldol or Thorazine, but may occur with other neuroleptics such as Compazine (a drug used to treat nausea).

Dystonia may occur unassociated with any other disease. It may affect only a single muscle, called focal dystonia. A common form of this is one that affects the sternocleidomastoid muscles, the muscles that turn the neck, resulting in a disorder called toritcollis. Another relatively common form of focal dystonia affects selected muscles of the forearm, resulting in an inability to write, called writer's cramp. Torticollis, writer's cramp, and other focal dystonias can be treated by injections of Botox. Dystonia may affect an entire group of muscles, called segmental dystonia, and rarely, it may affect most of the muscles in the body and is called generalized dystonia. Generalized dystonia usually starts in childhood and is inherited.

The terms Parkinson-plus disorder (Parkinson disease plus other symptoms), Parkinson-like disorder, Parkinson Syndrome, or Parkinsonism are applied to those disorders that initially resemble PD.

24. What is the difference between Parkinson disease and Parkinsonism?

The diagnosis of PD is made on the basis of the presence of the four cardinal symptoms, but these symptoms are not exclusive to PD. There are several disorders that even to an expert may initially be diagnosed as PD. The terms Parkinson-plus disorder (Parkinson disease plus other symptoms), Parkinson-like disorder, Parkinson Syndrome, or Parkinsonism are applied to those disorders that initially resemble PD.

On post-mortem examination of PD patients, the loss of dopamine cells in the substantia nigra is accompanied by a marker present in most of the dying cells. This marker is found in a part of the cell called the cytoplasm. Under the microscope it appears as a round body, almost filling the cell. It is called a Lewy body, after Friedrich Lewy, the doctor who first described it. How the Lewy body is formed, whether it is a sign of death or recovery, and the composition of the Lewy body are questions which science is seeking to answer.

As noted earlier, at birth we have 400,000 neurons in the substantia nigra, 200,000 on each side. The first symptoms of PD appear when there is a 60% loss of dopamine neurons. In the PD-like disorders, there may be an equal or greater loss of dopamine neurons, which explains in part why these disorders are less responsive to levodopa. In PD, if levodopa is started early and used in relatively high doses, it results in dyskinesias: abnormal involuntary movements and chaotic dance-like movements called chorea, all of which are worse on the side of the body more affected by PD. However, in the PD-like disorders, levodopa does not result in dyskinesias.

We know that PD both starts and progresses slowly— from diagnosis to need for treatment may be one or two years. However, the PD-like disorders start and progress more rapidly, with less time from diagnosis to treatment.

Corticobasilar degeneration (CBD) and **progressive supranuclear palsy (PSP)** are two Parkinson-like disorders characterized by a loss of neurons in the substantia nigra. However, the dying neurons do not contain Lewy bodies, as they do in PD. Instead, the dying neurons contain tangles of a protein called "tau." These tangles have a distinct appearance under a microscope. In CBD and PSP, in addition to the death of substantia nigra neurons, target neurons in the putamen and globus pallidus also die. This explains why CBD and PSP do not usually respond to levodopa.

Corticobasilar degeneration (CBD)

A movement disorder with rigidity symptoms similar to those of PD.

Progressive supranuclear palsy (PSP)

A movement disorder with symptoms similar to PD.

CBD may start asymmetrically (on one side), usually the right side. The right hand becomes rigid and the rigidity has a peculiar quality, called gegenhalten—it increases the more you move your hand. Sometimes the arm or hand does not do what you want it to do, as though it won't obey you. You arm is not weak or slow, it just won't do what you want. This is called a disconnection syndrome, or an "alien hand." CBD progresses more slowly than the other PD-like disorders. It may start with a loss of balance and falls and may resemble PSP.

Progressive supranuclear palsy (PSP) gets its name from the degeneration of centers in the brain that are located above (supra) the nuclei (groups of neurons) that control eye-movements. In PSP, you're unable to move your eyes, not because there's something wrong with your eye muscles, but because the **supra nuclear** centers are paralyzed (or palsied). The inability to move the eyes, first in an up-and-down direction, then in a side-to-side direction, usually appears early and enables a neurologist to make the diagnosis. If the eye movements are involved late, the diagnosis is more difficult and may be confused with PD. A specialist will test your eyes' ability to follow figures or lines on a tape that is past them. Normally in following the tape your eyes beat rapidly, a response called opticokinetic nystagmus (OKN), the absence of which, in one or more directions, suggest PSP. PSP is also characterized by the early appearance of postural instability with falls, difficulty with speaking and swallowing, and a poor response to levodopa. In some patients, an MRI reveals shrinkage of the brainstem. Although there's no specific treatment for PSP, a neurologist can suggest ways to minimize falls, improve swallowing, and make life more comfortable.

Supra nuclear

A neurologic disorder of unknown origin that gradually destroys cells in many areas of the brain, leading to serious and permanent problems.

Multiple-system atrophy (MSA) is the most common of the PD-like disorders. There are three forms of MSA. The first, **Shy-Drager**, or MSA with ANS involvement, may initially resemble PD. The absence of tremor, early and prominent symptoms of ANS insufficiency: dizziness on standing, difficulty swallowing, difficulty urinating, anterocollis (a flexed head), a relative lack of response to levodopa, and more rapid progression than PD, usually allows a neurologist to distinguish between the two. Proper management of the symptoms of ANS insufficiency can greatly improve a patient's quality of life. **MSA with ataxia** is a combination, in effect, of MSA with atrophy of the cerebellum. It can usually be distinguished from PD by the early appearance of postural instability (lack of balance), a voice that is difficult to understand, and a marked tremor of both hands that's present on movement and absent at rest. An MRI may reveal shrinkage of the cerebellum. **Striatonigral degeneration (SND)** is the most difficult of the MSAs to distinguish from PD. The early appearance of a flexed neck and a poor response to levodopa eventually leads to the diagnosis. Proper understanding of MSA often leads to a better quality of life. Unlike PD, the MSAs do not respond to deep brain stimulation (discussed later).

Dopa responsive dystonia (DRD) was first described in Japan by Professor Segawa and is often called Segawa's disease. DRD is an inherited disorder that starts in the teens, 20s, and 30s. It resembles PD except for the presence of prominent dystonia that may involve the neck, arms, legs, or trunk with accompanying tremor. DRD differs from other dystonias by its dramatic response to levodopa and differs from PD by its slower progression. DRD results from an inability to change the small amount of levodopa in the diet to dopamine because a

---

Tell Me More

Multiple-system atrophy (MSA)

A set of movement disorders with PD-like symptoms.

Shy-Drager

Multi-System Atrophy with ANS involvement

MSA with ataxia

A combination of MSA and atrophy of the cerebellum.

Striatonigral degeneration (SND)

The most difficult of the MSAs to distinguish from PD characterized by early appearance of a flexed neck and a poor response to levodopa.

Dopa responsive dystonia (DRD)

An inherited disorder that starts in the teens, 20s and 30s first described in Japan by Professor Segawa, often called Segawa's disease.

chemical, tetrahydrobiopterin, is missing in the brain. This can be overcome by giving levodopa in amounts comparable to those used in PD. Difficulty arises in distinguishing PD with dystonia from DRD, although PD with dystonia is not inherited and usually starts at a later age. A **PET scan** or a SPECT scan may distinguish DRD from PD and PD with dystonia, as the DRD PET-scan will not reveal a deficiency of dopamine, as in PD, in fact it will be normal.

PET scan

See Positron emission tomography.

Wilson disease is an inherited disorder in which a mutation in a gene on chromosome 13 leads to a deficiency in a protein called **ceruloplasmin**, which carries copper in the body. A deficiency in ceruloplasmin results in an excess of copper in the blood that, in turn, results in deposits of copper in the liver, the eyes, and the brain. Patients with Wilson disease develop symptoms at an early age, below age 40, and depending on where their copper has deposited they may have symptoms of a failing liver, psychiatric symptoms, chorea or Parkinsonism. PD patients who have a suspected family history of PD and whose symptoms develop at an early age should be examined for Wilson disease. The examination includes tests of liver function, a ceruloplasmin level, a blood and urine copper level, an examination by an ophthalmologist for copper deposits in the eyes and an MRI. Although Wilson disease is rare, one patient with Wilson disease for 1,000 patients with PD, the diagnosis should be pursued because there are specific treatments for Wilson disease.

Wilson disease

An inherited disorder in which a mutation in a gene on chromosome 13 leads to a deficiency in a protein called ceruloplasmin.

Ceruloplasmin

A protein which carries copper in the body.

25. Does having a tremor mean I have Parkinson disease?

Tremor is an involuntary oscillation of a group of muscles resulting in movement of an arm or a leg. In tremor, each oscillation resembles the previous one:

they are rhythmical. However, the frequency and amplitude of tremors differ from disease to disease. Tremors can be classified as *mild* (fine and barely noticeable), *mild-to-moderate* (noticeable but intermittent), *moderate* (noticeable and present most of the time), or *marked* (high amplitude and present most of the time). Some of the Parkinson-like disorders discussed in Question 24 involve tremors. *Essential tremor (ET)*, a hyper-kinetic disorder, is actually the most common movement disorder—in fact it is 20 times more common than PD. However, fewer than 2% of people with ET have symptoms sufficiently disabling to require treatment.

The tremor of ET can usually, but not always, be distinguished from the tremor of PD. Generally, the tremor of ET starts in both hands simultaneously, while the tremor of PD usually starts in only one hand. The tremor of ET is a sustention or postural tremor, a tremor that appears when you hold your hands in front of you, contracting the muscles of your forearm while maintaining (or sustaining) a posture. ET is also an action, or kinetic, tremor; a tremor that appears when you move or use your hands. Initially ET can be bothersome or embarrassing, but not disabling. However, after several years, ET may become disabling and impair or limit such everyday activities as dressing, feeding, shaving, and writing. Although a postural or sustention tremor is characteristic of ET, a similar tremor occurs in 20% of PD patients. In PD, the postural tremor begins in one hand. PD patients can have both a resting and a postural tremor. Such a tremor is called a complex or compound tremor. When a sustention tremor appears in one hand, with no other symptoms of PD, it may be difficult to predict whether the tremor will evolve into PD or ET. In some people

Tremors can be classified as mild (fine and barely noticeable), mild-to-moderate (noticeable but intermittent), moderate (noticeable and present most of the time), or marked (high amplitude and present most of the time).

Tell Me More

ET evolves into PD, and in some families there are people with ET, people with PD, and people with ET and PD. At present, however, there is not enough data to say whether ET and PD are related.

Physiologic tremor

Is the tremor that is present in everyone, brought out with stress, a fever, or with an overactive thyroid gland.

Physiologic tremor is the tremor that is present in everyone, the tremor that is brought out with stress, a fever, or with an over-active thyroid gland. The tremor of ET and physiological tremor are thought to arise from over-activity of a "tremor circuit" in a region of the brain below the basal ganglia. Many experts believe ET is an exaggerated form of physiological tremor, one that does not go away. Others believe ET and physiological tremor are separate and distinct.

One or two drinks of alcohol may help ET, presumably by suppressing the tremor circuit. However, alcohol usually does not help the tremor of PD. A word of caution: alcohol overuse or abuse can, in time, aggravate ET. And withdrawal from alcohol after heavy drinking can itself result in a tremor: alcoholic withdrawal tremor. Whether the tremor of alcohol abuse or alcohol withdrawal is a separate tremor or an exaggeration of a physiological tremor or of ET is unknown at present.

Dystonic tremor refers to a tremor that appears in a hand, leg, or neck that is dystonic: a disorder in which a muscle or group of muscles is abnormally or over-contracted, the tone is increased, and movement is compromised. While one set of muscles is contracted, the opposing muscles are also contracted, instead of relaxing, as though your muscles are "fighting" each other. Dystonic tremor is task-specific: it appears when you attempt a specific task such as writing, playing a musical instrument, throwing a baseball, or putting in golf (where it may be called the "yips"). It is as though the particular task has become "over-learned" and cannot be performed when you want to perform it. Dystonic tremor may occur independently of other disorders or, rarely, it may appear as part of PD. The treatment of dystonic tremor is injection of Botox into the over-contracted muscles.

Tremor may also be caused by several disorders or drugs. Such a tremor is thought to be an exaggeration of the normal physiologic tremor resulting from over-activity of the tremor circuit. The tremor is bilateral, in both hands, and is a postural, sustention, or action tremor, not a resting tremor, nor is it associated with rigidity or bradykinesia. The tremor is associated with other symptoms of the disorder, or is time-related to the start of the tremor-causing drug. The tremor disappears when the disorder is treated or after the offending drug is stopped. Among the more common drugs that cause tremors are:

- Amiodarone or Cordarone—used to regulate the heartbeat
- Dolbutamine—used in the hospital to maintain blood pressure and blood flow
- Ephedrine and Phenylephrine—nasal decongestants
- Haloperidol or Haldol—used to control abnormal behavior such as schizophrenia
- Lidocaine—a local anesthetic drug also used in the hospital to regulate the heartbeat
- Lithium—used to treat bipolar disorder
- Metoclopramide or Reglan—used to regulate gastric motility
- Valproic acid or Depakote—an anti-seizure drug used to treat epilepsy and bipolar disorder

26. What is a hyperkinetic movement disorder?

Some movement disorders involve increased movement and are termed hyperkinetic movement disorders. **Tics** and tremors fit this category, as do akathisia, chorea, and myoclonus. **Akathisia** is an inner sense of restlessness, like an "ants in the pants" feeling. It may complicate levodopa treatment of PD or treatment of some psychiatric disorders by selective serotonin reuptake inhibitors (SSRIs), anti-seizure drugs, or neuroleptic drugs.

Chorea, or dyskinesia, is a slow (one or two beats per second), moderate amplitude, non-rhythmical, chaotic, dance-like, flowing movement involving the head and neck (separately or together), tongue, arms and legs. Chorea can occur in Huntington disease (an inherited disorder of the brain), in PD treatment with levodopa, during psychiatric treatment with neuroleptic drugs, during pregnancy, during treatment with phenytoin or Dilantin (anti-seizure drugs), after strokes of the basal ganglia, in hypoglycemia (low blood sugar), hypothyroidism (overactive thyroid), liver failure, and in Wilson disease.

Myoclonus is a contraction of a muscle or group of muscles lasting less than 0.3 seconds. Myoclonus can be of moderate to high amplitude, can involve a single part of the body (an arm or leg) called focal myoclonus, or can be a coordinated, synchronized rhythmical movement of an arm and a leg, both arms, both legs (called segmental myoclonus), or both arms and legs and the trunk (called generalized myoclonus). It can also result from a sudden relaxation of a group of muscles which causes the limb to suddenly jerk. This relaxation is called asterixis and may complicate liver failure.

Tics

Involuntary muscle twitches or movements.

Akathisia

An inner sense of restlessness, like an "ants in the pants" feeling.

Chorea

Movement disorders characterized by dance-like, flowing movements of arms or legs, often involving every part of the body. Also called dyskinesia.

Myoclonus

A movement disorder that consists of quick, jerking movements that can involve one finger or the entire body.

Myoclonus can arise from an electrical discharge in the cortex (as part of an epileptic seizure), in the basal ganglia, and in the spinal cord. It can occur as a normal phenomenon as when you are falling asleep, waking up, or when you are startled. Hiccoughs are myoclonus of your diaphragm. Myoclonus may be triggered by a variety of stimuli including light, sound, and sudden fright. Like chorea, myoclonus can be caused by a variety of disorders, including Alzheimer's disease, AIDS, Creutzfeldt-Jakob disease, brain damage in utero, and circulatory failure as in cardiac arrest. Nocturnal myoclonus, which occurs while you fall asleep or awaken from sleep, may be aggravated by levodopa in PD patients.

27. What do I do after I've been diagnosed with Parkinson disease?

If you've been diagnosed with PD, you may feel many conflicting emotions. You may fear becoming physically, emotionally, and economically dependent on others or you may worry because the money that you've saved for retirement may have to go toward paying your medical expenses. You may think that you no longer control your future or that you're alone— isolated. All of these concerns are worrisome but normal. And there are things you can and should do to take control of PD.

Your first reaction may be denial. You may wonder whether the diagnosis is correct. Such a reaction gives you time to digest the news and formulate a response. "Nobody in my family has it," you say. "I'm sure it's stress. If I rearrange my schedule, exercise regularly, pay attention to what I eat, and get a good night of sleep, my symptoms will go away." Although exercise, nutrition, stress management, and rest are important,

If you've been diagnosed with PD, you may feel many conflicting emotions. You may fear becoming physically, emotionally, and economically dependent on others or you may worry because the money that you've saved for retirement may have to go toward paying your medical expenses.

they won't cure PD. Or your first reaction may be relief that your problem isn't a brain tumor or a stroke and that it's not your imagination, as you've known that something was wrong.

Your second reaction may be fear and anxiety. Realizing that you have PD can make you fearful and anxious. You and your family have no idea what to expect—thus, you think the worst. You may fear losing your job, your friends, and most of all, your independence. These are honest reasons for being fearful or anxious; however, an excellent way to master fear is to learn as much as you can about PD. Talk with people who have PD and who have gone through similar experiences. They can tell you what worked—or what didn't. Find resources, information, workshops, and support groups that can help you to understand PD. For example, National Parkinson Foundation has more than 1,000 support groups throughout the United States and has an Internet page (www.parkinson.org) where you can ask questions about PD. The Muhammad Ali Parkinson Center also has a large outreach program where you can get help.

If fear and anxiety aren't recognized, they'll show up as hostility and resentment. You may wonder what you have done to deserve PD. Your anger may be directed at the people you love. You may snap at minor slights or disappointments. If this happens, stop, think, and do the following:

Recognize that having PD does not excuse being angry with others. Facing the reasons for behavior is the beginning of self-awareness, and self-awareness is the first step in coping with, adjusting to, and eventually controlling PD.

Understand that loved ones are also upset because you have PD and are trying to be supportive, although they don't know how. Don't be afraid to tell them what you need or to talk about it. Everyone will benefit. Learn healthy ways to channel anger. Talk honestly and frankly with your spouse, a friend, or a counselor. Start by connecting with the people around you. For example, if you hesitate or "freeze" while walking, people may be puzzled. Rather than being angry, hostile, or resentful when they stare, say this: "I have PD, and occasionally I get stuck and can't move; it'll pass in a few minutes."

Your third reaction may be depression. Sadness, despair, and helplessness often follow anger and resentment, especially if unrecognized. These are symptoms of **depression**, which is common in PD. If you find yourself crying frequently, withdrawing from day-to-day activities, or sleeping too much or too little, you may be depressed. Seek help because treatments are available. A risk in accepting help for the physical aspects of your PD is that you'll become dependent on others. To lessen this, retain as much responsibility for yourself as you can. By doing as much as you can independently, you'll feel better about yourself.

Understand that loved ones are also upset because you have PD and are trying to be supportive, although they don't know how. Don't be afraid to tell them what you need or to talk about it.

Tell Me More

Depression

Chronic feelings of sadness, despair, and helplessness.

PART THREE

Things You Should Know

Why does Parkinson disease get worse?

What is freezing of gait (FOG)?

Why am I having difficulty swallowing?

More . . .

28. What does it mean that Parkinson disease is a progressive disease?

Parkinson disease is considered a progressive disorder because it changes with time; its initial symptoms may worsen and new symptoms may appear. The new symptoms may include postural hypotension (a drop in blood pressure on sitting or standing), freezing of gait (FOG), falls, swallowing difficulty, and weight loss. The new symptoms may include anxiety, depression, and forgetfulness. Some of these symptoms result from the drugs used to treat PD, but most result from PD.

The earliest symptoms of PD can be so subtle and vague as to be dismissed or taken for something else. When you look back you can see that symptoms you thought were related to aging were actually part of PD.

The earliest symptoms of PD can be so subtle and vague as to be dismissed or taken for something else. When you look back you can see that symptoms you thought were related to aging were actually part of PD. When PD begins, usually only one side is affected and, as PD progresses, the other side is involved. Often, you are aware of the symptoms, but don't think anything is wrong—it may be your spouse who insists there is a change.

PD affects the basal ganglia, which are situated at the base of the brain between the cortex (the thinking brain) and the brainstem and spinal cord (the parts controlling movement). The cortex specifies the speed, amplitude, and duration of movement. The basal ganglia translate these commands into movements that occur without your awareness of them, movements such as swinging your arms while walking. Because the movements are automatic, many PD patients do not realize they are slowed. The basal ganglia function like both the accelerator and brake in a car. The substantia nigra, putamen, and caudate nucleus comprise the accelerator; the "gasoline" is dopamine; and the globus pallidus, subthalamic nucleus, and thalamus comprise the brakes. In PD, not only is your accelerator defective, resulting in slowing down, but it is as though your brakes are always on, thus slowing you down even further.

29. Why does Parkinson disease get worse?

PD worsens mainly due to increased cell death—the process is explained in this section. There are 100 billion neurons in the brain. For each nerve cell there are, perhaps, 10 times as many support cells, called glial cells, which bring oxygen and needed chemicals to the nerve cells. All cells in the body, including the brain, have parts called organelles. The cell's organelles include the nucleus, the "brain" of the cell, which contains the cell's DNA (genes).

Neurons are designed to perform specific tasks by their genes, but are vulnerable to dying. There are a few ways in which neurons die: they can be killed by infectious agents such as viruses; they can be killed by toxins such as iron, calcium, manganese, and nitrous oxide; or they can be killed by a lack of oxygen (or too much oxygen). Nerve cells can also "commit suicide:" they can initiate suicide programs that are built into all cells. These programs, called apoptosis, are partly controlled by genes and partly by outside agents. This has been one of the popular theories as to why neurons die, but recent studies have moved away from apoptosis as a cause of cell death in PD.

Whether cells are killed by an infection or a toxin, are genetically vulnerable, or commit suicide, much research focuses on the mitochondria—the "power plants" of the cells. Mitochondria vary in number from a few dozen to several thousand, depending on the cell and its requirement for energy. Mitochondria mainly die from either a lack of nutrients or a lack of replacement parts. As they extract energy from food molecules, such as fats and sugars, they use oxygen to produce a basic chemical fuel called ATP, the "gasoline," so to speak, that powers most of the cell's activity. There are carriers called complexes in the mitochondria that use oxygen dissolved in the cell to extract energy from fats and sugars. Different carriers are derived from some of the B vitamins.

In humans, 100% of your mitochondria come from your mother, as only mitochondria and their genes are passed along to the fertilized egg. The mitochondrial genes are more stable and less susceptible to variation than the genes in the nucleus of the cell. The process of generating energy in the cell, like the process of generating energy for industry, results in the production of toxic products, or pollutants. Like industry, the cell must remove the pollutants so that its environment, especially the environment inside and outside the mitochondria, isn't poisoned. The toxic products produced inside the mitochondria are reactive chemical species called free radicals, and have the ability to attack the normal components of the cell.

Antioxidants are chemicals that "neutralize" free radicals and play a major role in protecting the mitochondria and the rest of the cell. The antioxidants consist of a series of enzymes, each specific for a specific free radical. The work of the enzyme is helped by additional scavengers of free radicals such as Vitamins C and E, glutathione, and Coenzyme Q10. If the free radical scavengers fail and free radicals increase inside the cell, changes in proteins such as alpha synuclein may occur, causing it to aggregate and clump, altering its function and resulting in death. The death of the cell by apoptosis is required to destroy cells that represent a threat to the integrity of the body, such as cells infected with viruses. It is unclear whether this process is relevant to the cell death associated with progression of PD.

30. Does iron worsen Parkinson disease?

Adults store one to three grams of iron in their bodies (about 1/10 ounce), which is maintained through a balance between dietary intake and loss. After iron is absorbed, it is bound to a circulating protein called transferrin, which attaches to receptors on specific cells such as the substantia nigra neurons and is carried into the cell. After binding to the receptor on the cell's surface, transferrin is taken into the cell where it detaches itself from the receptor and releases the iron where it binds and is stored for later use. As the pigmented granules disappear, iron is released into the cell and, alone or attached to other molecules, acts as a free radical. There are some researchers who believe that rasagiline, a drug that blocks a specific enzyme called MAO-B, may among other mechanisms remove (chelate) the excess iron in the cell and that this may slow the progression of PD.

31. How can free radicals worsen Parkinson disease?

Molecules are composed of atoms bonded together, which is accomplished by the sharing of electrons. When two atoms come together and their electrons pair up, a bond is created. Such electron pairs are stable; nearly 100% of all electrons in the body exist in a paired state. When a chemical bond between two atoms is broken, the electrons can stay with one atom or the other, or they can split up. If one atom captures both electrons it will develop a negative charge, while the other atom will develop a positive charge. Both of these charged atoms are now free radicals.

The forces that disrupt chemical bonds include radiation such as ultraviolet light, infra-red rays, radiation from the earth's core, and cosmic rays. The disruptive forces also include other chemicals, termed toxins. Among these toxins are gases (carbon monoxide, manganese fumes, ozone), chemicals (arsenic, cyanide, mercury), substances released by invading bacteria and fungi, and chemicals generated in your cells, especially in your mitochondria. The resulting free radicals may have short or long existences; some can last a lifetime, many exist for less than five seconds, and some for only a hundredth of a microsecond.

The forces that disrupt chemical bonds include radiation such as ultraviolet light, infra-red rays, radiation from the earth's core, and cosmic rays. The disruptive forces also include other chemicals, termed toxins.

To appreciate the importance of free radicals and to understand the magnitude of the change they produce in each of your 100 billion neurons, it is only necessary to cut an apple and expose it to air. The iron in the apple interacts with oxygen in the air and the apple "rusts." It's disconcerting to think so, but something similar happens when the iron, stored as co-factors for vital enzymes in our cells, and the fat that composes the vital membranes of our cells, are exposed to reactive oxygen species. In each of the 100 billion neurons in our brain, and each of the 20 to 1,000 mitochondria in each neuron, a constant struggle is waged every second between the cell's need to generate energy and its vulnerability to the toxic products created by this need.

Numerous antioxidants are marketed as nutritional supplements, and naturally people wonder which antioxidant is best or most powerful. Technically, if it were known that one antioxidant was more selective for a particular free radical, and that the particular antioxidant could readily reach the cell, enter it and inactivate the free radical, then an antioxidant as "a guided missile" could be delivered to the cell. Unfortunately, at present, we lack such a "guided missile." In trying to devise a rational scheme for their use, research has focused on those antioxidants that play a role in the efficient functioning of the mitochondria, the power plants of the cell. Among the most promising are the following:

The "B" Vitamins. Although they are not antioxidants, they are needed for operation of the citric acid cycle and the electron transport system. B vitamins include thiamin (B-1), riboflavin (B-2), niacin (B-3), pantothenic acid (B-5), pyridoxine (B-6), biotin (B-7), and cyanocobalamin (B-12). Folic acid and vitamin B-12 are needed for a healthy nervous system. A combination of vitamin B-6, folic acid and vitamin B-12 reduces homocysteine levels. Homocysteine, an amino acid, may be a risk factor for heart attack and stroke, and may be increased in PD patients on levodopa/carbidopa. As vitamin B-6, in doses of 50 mg or more per day, may decrease the absorption of levodopa, B-complex vitamins should be taken at night, 4 hours between the last and the next dose of levodopa/carbidopa.

Vitamins C and E. Vitamin C is a major antioxidant. It may be especially effective against the highly reactive free radicals generated by oxygen and by metals such as copper, iron, and manganese. Vitamin E is a fat-soluble vitamin that may be especially effective against the highly reactive free radicals generated by oxygen that attack the lipid layers of cell membranes.

Coenzyme Q10. Coenzyme Q10 is an antioxidant within the mitochondria that neutralizes many of the toxic free radicals generated by the normal functioning of the mitochondria. In doses of 1,200-2,400 mg per day, Coenzyme Q10 may slow the progression of PD. This is suggested by a single small study that is in the process of being corroborated.

Glutathione. Glutathione, a tripeptide, is a major intracellular antioxidant found in high concentrations inside nigral neurons. As PD progresses and the nigral neurons die, the concentration of glutathione decreases. It's unknown at this time if this is a cause or a consequence of PD.

Alpha lipoic acid and *acetyl L carnitine* are antioxidants that "soak up" free radicals generated by the citrus acid cycle. In addition, alpha lipoic acid can chelate iron and copper to a degree, although there is no real proof that either antioxidant is helpful in treating PD.

32. What is the role of fat in the diet of people with PD?

There's evidence that fatty acids, derived from dietary fat, may play a role in the progression of PD. Scientific studies indicate that the risk of developing PD is higher in people who eat saturated (animal) fat than those who eat polyunsaturated (fish) fat. Thus, the prevalence of PD is one third lower in Japan, a fish-eating nation, than in America, a meat-eating nation.

Decreased saturated and increased polyunsaturated fats play a major role in slowing, halting, and preventing atherosclerosis, heart attack and stroke. Regulation of dietary fat may play a similar role in slowing or halting PD. Evidence suggests that inflammation, the result of an over-production of "bad" versus "good" omega 3

Decreased saturated and increased polyunsaturated fats play a major role in slowing, halting, and preventing atherosclerosis, heart attack and stroke. Regulation of dietary fat may play a similar role in slowing or halting PD.

fats may be responsible for the atherosclerotic plaques that clog arteries, resulting in heart attack and stroke.

The brain is 60% fat but, unlike the body where fat is mainly a source of energy, fat in the brain forms the outer membranes of the one hundred billion neurons, or brain cells. It is thought that Lewy bodies may have defective fatty membranes, containing the wrong ratio of "good" to "bad" fats and, because the cell's membranes are not solid walls, toxic substances might leak back into the cell and destroy it.

The source of "good" or omega 3 fats are the fatty acids called EPA and DHA. Fatty fish such as herring, mackerel, salmon, sardines, and tuna are rich in omega 3 fatty acids. However, some of these fish have, concentrated in their fat, toxins such as mercury. As a rule herring, salmon, and sardines have lower levels of mercury than other fatty fish.

Changing to a diet higher in polyunsaturated and lower in saturated fatty acids, rich in essential fatty acids, and balanced toward omega-3/omega-6 fatty acids decreases the risk of death from heart attack and stroke. By decreasing inflammation, such a diet may also be helpful in slowing the progression of PD. Patients recently diagnosed with PD should consider adopting a diet lower in saturated fat and higher in polyunsaturated fats: a "heart and stroke friendly" diet, as well as taking fish oil in doses of at least 1 gram three times a day.

33. What is freezing of gait (FOG)?

Freezing of gait (FOG) is a common symptom in advanced PD—PD that's been diagnosed for at least five years. It occurs in 30% of PD patients with advanced PD, though it can also occur early in PD and may be one of the initial symptoms. FOG is characterized by "start hesitation" or "failure of gait initiation," meaning the inability to start walking. FOG also occurs when you turn, or when you think about turning. Suddenly you get stuck, your feet can't move, as though they're glued to the floor or held there by magnets, and you're frozen like a statue—hence the name freezing of gait. FOG can occur when you come to a doorway or even think about coming to a doorway, when you come to a curb or think about coming to a curb. FOG may be accompanied by **anteropulsion** (a feeling of being pushed forward) or **retropulsion** (a feeling of being pulled backward). It may be preceded by short, shuffling steps. FOG is often accompanied by postural instability, a feeling of being unbalanced. Common to all the situations that result in FOG is a change in your stride length and/or your stride velocity (or the thought of changing your stride length or velocity). It's as though you want to do something, but your feet don't like what you are doing (or thinking) and they refuse to move.

Starting to walk is like starting your car by turning on your engine, pumping your acceleration and releasing your brake. In start hesitation, it's as though your brake can't be released. In turning, approaching a doorway, or walking in a crowded room, your stride length and/or stride velocity must change. This is like taking your foot off your accelerator and pushing down on your brake. In FOG it's as though your brake locks and you can't release it. FOG can be helped, in part, by learning "tricks," much like jiggling with your brakes to get you started or to get you going again. Among the "tricks" that work in some patients and that we teach at the Muhammad Ali Parkinson Clinic are the following:

Anteropulsion

A feeling of being pushed forward.

Retropulsion

The need to take steps backward in order to begin moving forward.

Teach yourself to step over a real or imagined line or lines on the floor to get yourself going. Somehow, parallel lines drawn on the floor, or imagined as being drawn on the floor, "trick" your feet into obeying your brain.

Carry a laser light, or a cane fitted with a laser light. Shine it on the floor and step over it, again, to get yourself going. Note: this trick doesn't work in bright sunshine.

Carry a cane or a walking stick and tap it on the floor in synch with a tune you're humming as you walk. Somehow, this combined visual and auditory trick allows your feet to continue walking even as you change your stride length and/or velocity.

Hum a tune, or snap your fingers, to start walking or to continue walking as you change your stride length and/or velocity.

Chant a phrase such as "Go, Go, Go," or "Turn, Turn, Turn," to start walking or to continue walking.

If FOG occurs early, before you're started on anti-Parkinson drugs, it will usually improve when you add a dopamine agonist (Mirapex, or Neupro, or Requip), an MAO-B inhibitor such as Azilect or Zelapar, amantadine, or levodopa/carbidopa. If FOG occurs after you've been started on levodopa/carbidopa, then adding a dopamine agonist, an MAO-B inhibitor, amantadine, entacapone (Comtan), or tolcapone (Tasmar) may help. If FOG occurs after you've been started on a dopamine agonist, then adding an MAO-B inhibitor, amantadine, or levodopa/carbidopa may help.

If FOG occurs after you've been on levodopa/carbidopa, try to determine if it occurs when the levodopa/carbidopa is working or when it is not. At the Muhammad Ali Parkinson Clinic, we ask patients who suffer from FOG to visit us in the morning, after they've stopped levodopa/carbidopa for at least 16 hours. We examine them and determine how often FOG occurs, then give them a dose of levodopa/carbidopa and examine them after an hour. This allows us to determine what effect the medication has on FOG. We may then recommend additional levodopa/carbidopa or adding entacapone or tolcapone.

34. Why do I fall?

Falling and loss of balance occur in people with PD and can result in major injuries: fractured shoulders, hips, ankles, and even skulls. To decrease falling, it helps to understand why you lose your balance and fall. Falls result from postural instability or loss of "righting reflexes:" the ability to right yourself and take measures to prevent a fall. Thus, if you trip or are pushed, by the time you realize it, your righting reflexes have changed the position of your head, neck, trunk, arms, and legs so that you either avert the fall or cushion yourself if you do fall.

Your eyes are less important in righting yourself than the sensors in your feet or those in your inner ears.

The righting reflexes are alerted to your changed position (sense of "falling through space") by sensors in your feet (position sense), inner ears, and by your eyes. The alerting information from your feet and inner ears travels to a region of your brain called the thalamus. Your eyes are less important in righting yourself than the sensors in your feet or those in your inner ears. Thus, a blind man can right himself and not fall after he trips. A person with impaired sensors in his feet or inner ears is less likely to right himself and more likely to fall after tripping. The information sent to the thalamus is acted upon, enabling your cerebellum to try to avert the fall by ordering several rapid adjustments in muscle tone. In PD, these adjustments may not be rapid enough to prevent a fall.

In PD, because of the decreased ability to right yourself when you trip and a decreased ability to maintain your balance when you stand, the following advice may be helpful:

Avoid snow, ice, wet or slippery surfaces. When you slip on ice, the change in your body's position is more rapid than when you trip on a dry surface. The messages signaling the change in your position reach your cerebellum and thalamus quicker and there is less time for you to react, so you are more likely to fall.

Avoid uneven or hilly surfaces—these result in the position sensors in your feet and inner ears bombarding your vestibular nuclei with messages, one after the other, each telling of a change in direction, position, or velocity of your legs. This bombardment may overwhelm your ability to respond and you're more likely to fall.

Avoid walking in the dark. Your brain also senses the environment through your eyes. In the dark, you depend on the position sensors in your feet and inner ears; they are your "fall back" systems. If, as may happen, one of these systems fails, you are likely to fall in the dark.

35. Why do I get dizzy?

Dizziness usually occurs in PD because of orthostatic or postural hypotension (a drop in blood pressure on sitting or standing). To understand why your blood pressure drops, you must understand hypertension or high blood pressure. Your brain and heart need a constant flow of blood, a constant cardiac output, under all conditions: lying down, sitting, and standing. Your brain demands 30% of your cardiac output, and your heart about 20%. If your brain does not get its 30%, it shuts down and you black out.

We cannot easily measure blood flow, but we can measure blood pressure. As you grow older, your arteries narrow and their resistance increases. To maintain 30% of blood flow to your brain, your blood pressure must increase to compensate for the increased arterial resistance. In PD, orthostatic hypotension results from an inability of a faulty autonomic nervous system (ANS) to constrict your arteries when you sit or stand. Orthostatic hypotension occurs in about 20% of PD patients, and almost all patients with MSA.

When you lie down, your head and your heart are at the same level, so your heart does not have to work hard to pump blood to your brain. When you sit, your head is above your heart, and your heart has to work harder. In part, your heart works harder by beating faster, and in part you constrict your blood vessels. However, if you can't constrict your blood vessels or your heart can't beat faster—your brain will get less blood and you'll feel dizzy or faint. Likewise, when you stand after sitting, fluid (the equivalent of two units of blood) is redistributed from your chest and abdomen to your legs. To accommodate the larger volume of distribution, your heart has to work harder to pump blood to your brain. Again, your heart works harder by beating faster and constricting your blood vessels.

The following letter from a woman whose husband has MSA illustrates what you can do to manage orthostatic hypotension. If she can do it—so can you.

My husband was diagnosed with MSA. The symptoms that are most difficult to deal with are his orthostatic and postprandial hypotension (decreased blood pressure after eating). His postprandial hypotension is more dramatic because it causes his blood pressure to crash after he eats, which often results in his passing out. His orthostatic hypotension results in balance problems and falling, as well as in his passing out.

Note that after you eat a standard sized meal, 30% of your blood supply goes to your stomach. This puts an even greater demand on your heart if you stand: 30% of your blood must go to your brain, but 30% is already going to your stomach. If you have orthostatic hypotension, lie down after you eat, especially after a large meal.

I take my husband's blood pressure several times a day. It was through my discovery of lying him down and taking his blood pressure that I noticed it was always high (supine hypertension). I then discovered that if he passed out and I called "911" the paramedics would put him on a stretcher, which caused his blood pressure to increase. Thus by the time he arrived in the Emergency Room (ER) the doctor was treating his supine hypertension, and NOT his orthostatic hypotension. But when he returned home the orthostatic hypotension on sitting or standing became the problem—again. Through trial and error, I learned and convinced the doctors that, in addition to orthostatic hypotension, he also had supine hypertension.

We're between a rock and a hard place and so we've taken the approach, rightly or wrongly, that we prefer the high blood pressure over the low. With high pressure, the risk is theoretical: it's not immediate. With orthostatic hypotension the risk is real and immediate. We treat the low blood

Note that after you eat a standard sized meal, 30% of your blood supply goes to your stomach.

pressure with pressure stockings, adequate fluids and salt, fludrocortisones or Florinef (a volume expander), *midodrine or Proamatine* (a drug that simulates the action of norepinephrine), *and neostigmine* (a drug used in myasthenia gravis, but one that can prevent the development of orthostatic hypotension without provoking supine hypertension).

In addition to having orthostatic hypotension and supine hypertension, people with MSA (and some people with PD) can have bradycardia, a slow heart rate (fewer than 50 beats/minute). If you stand up and your blood pressure drops, your heart rate usually increases to maintain the same flow of blood to your brain. This is what prevents you from passing out. However, if, when your blood pressure drops, you can't increase your heart rate (because of a problem with your ANS), then you pass-out. The slow heart rate can be treated with a pacemaker. Although on occasion my husband's heart rate has slowed below 50 beats/minute, at this time we have decided NOT to have a pacemaker.

MSA has made me learn things I never wanted to know, but it has made me my husband's advocate. I check his blood pressure every morning when he gets out of bed; this is usually the time of his lowest pressure. He has learned NOT to jump out of bed, because his pressure drops dramatically. He first sits at the edge of his bed and dangles his legs. Then, with help, he slowly gets out of bed. If he's dizzy, and his pressure is too low, we put him back in bed, wait a few minutes and try again. Some days it takes several attempts before he's ready to stand and his blood pressure has adjusted to his standing position.

The bathroom is a problem. When a man stands and urinates, his blood pressure may drop as he empties his bladder. The faster he empties his bladder, the more his pressure drops.

If it drops too much, he can black out. This is called micturi-tion syncope. My husband has learned never to stand when he urinates and he has learned to urinate slowly.

My husband spends 30 minutes a day on a recumbent bicy-cle. On the bicycle, his head and heart are almost at the same level, so it's easier for his heart to pump blood to his head and he's less likely to black out while exercising. I give him midodrine, a drug that raises his pressure, an hour before he gets on the bicycle. The midodrine can minimize the drop in blood pressure that some MSA and PD patients experience when they exercise. He pedals slowly; this improves the tone of his muscles, important because it's the muscles that send blood from his veins to his heart. After he finishes with the bicycle, I massage his legs; I always start at his feet and massage upward, moving the fluid that has been trapped in his feet upward. The less fluid trapped in his legs, the more that is available to be pumped to his head.

A friend has a swimming pool and we use it three times a week. If the water is too warm, the blood vessels in his arms and legs dilate and he can black out because there's not enough blood to circulate and be pumped to his head. Because of this, we never go into a hot tub. If the water is too cold, the blood vessels in his legs constrict, his heart rate increases and he can black out from that as well. Walking in the pool is good; the pressure of the water forces the blood out of his feet and legs and into his circulation. My hus-band wears support hose. They are a pain to put on, but they prevent pooling of blood in his feet and legs.

My husband eats five small meals a day. Too much food all at once causes postprandial hypotension and he blacks out. He avoids coffee and tea because the caffeine is a diuretic; it makes him urinate and decreases his circulating fluid vol-ume. The caffeine can also speed up his heart rate.

My husband drinks 6 to 8 glasses of water a day. If he did not keep up with his fluids, he'd black out. Some MSA patients do NOT sweat, but my husband sweats profusely. He can lose a lot of fluid if he sweats, especially if it's hot. How much extra fluid does he drink? It's a guess. I weigh my husband every day. If he's losing weight (3 to 5 pounds in a day), his blood pressure is low, and his heart rate is fast, he needs more fluid (think dehydration). If he's gaining weight (3 to 5 pounds a day), his supine pressure is too high, and his legs are puffy, he needs less fluid.

I've learned not to use drugs called beta-blockers, such as propranolol (Inderal). Beta blockers are "wonder" drugs: they lower blood pressure, control rapid heart rates, decrease tremor (a problem in my husband), and relieve migraine headaches. But beta blockers dramatically drop his blood pressure. I've also learned not to use drugs called calcium channel blockers: drugs that dilate arteries and improve circulation. While I want to improve my husband's circulation, the calcium channel blockers can dramatically drop his blood pressure. My husband has learned NOT to drink alcohol. Alcohol dilates the blood pressure, and in my husband one drink is enough to cause him to black out. I know of people with MSA and PD who can and do drink in moderation. The watchword is caution.

36. Why do I have difficulty swallowing?

Swallowing difficulty (dysphagia) usually occurs late in PD, but may occur at any time and early on might be difficult to recognize. It can vary from mild (an inconvenience), to marked, resulting in significant weight loss. Some of the symptoms of difficulty swallowing include:

- Swallowing repeatedly after taking a bite
- Coughing and/or choking while eating (this results from food particles being swallowed into your

trachea and lungs, instead of your esophagus and stomach)

- Changing voice (swallowing and speaking share many of the same muscles so a disorder that affects your swallowing muscles is likely to affect your speaking muscles as well)
- Drooling (this results from difficulty swallowing your saliva)
- Eating slowly
- Weight loss (the most common reason for weight loss in PD is difficulty swallowing)

Swallowing requires the coordinated action of many muscles, both voluntary and smooth. First, your tongue and jaw muscles prepare the food to be swallowed by chewing it and mixing it with saliva. Then the muscles in the back of your mouth and throat start the swallow. They also seal off your windpipe and nose to keep food and liquids from backing up into them. Next, the muscles of your esophagus propel the food into your stomach. Slow or rigid muscles at any level can result in difficulty swallowing. The same slowness and rigidity that affects the muscles in your arms and legs affects the muscles in your throat.

Understanding the mechanics of swallowing and educating yourself about steps you can take to facilitate the process may decrease your difficulty swallowing. For instance, people with PD unknowingly tend to bend or flex their necks when they sit, forcing themselves to look down. This makes chewing and swallowing difficult because your jaw is at a mechanical disadvantage. However, raising your neck and chewing is much easier on your jaw muscles. One way to ensure this happens is to straddle your chair at meal times, which straightens your spine and forces you to look up. Another trick is to rest your elbows on the table, which will also straighten your neck and force you to look up. Lastly, if you have difficulty swallowing you can take your carbidopa/levodopa in the form of Parcopa, which dissolves in your mouth. Take the Parcopa one hour before you eat so that when you're ready to eat, the Parcopa will be at peak concentration and your muscles of chewing and swallowing will be at their best.

Swallowing difficulty is best evaluated by a speech therapist trained to evaluate disorders of speech and swallowing.

37. Why am I losing weight?

About 20% of people with PD lose weight, especially people with advanced PD. This weight loss can be marked, with patients losing 10–20% of their body weight over a short time (six months to a year). Before assuming the weight loss is from PD, you should be evaluated by your doctor for other causes of weight loss such as AIDS, diabetes, cancer, colitis, hyperthyroidism, kidney or liver disease, malabsorption, and tuberculosis. The weight loss in these disorders is like starvation: you break down and lose both fat and muscle, whereas in PD, you just break down fat. If your weight loss is thought to be related to PD, there are several reasons for it:

Decreased Appetite. Decreased appetite may be caused by anti-Parkinson drugs such as levodopa/carbidopa. This can usually be treated by supplementing each dose of levodopa/carbidopa with more carbidopa, which will decrease the nausea and loss of appetite that may accompany your treatment. Decreased appetite might be caused by loss of your sense of smell with a corresponding loss of sense of taste. This can usually

Before assuming the weight loss is from PD, you should be evaluated by your doctor for other causes of weight loss such as AIDS, diabetes, cancer, colitis, hyperthyroidism, kidney or liver disease, malabsorption, and tuberculosis.

be treated by using condiments and spices to make your food more appealing.

Anxiety and/or Depression. If you're anxious or depressed you may lose your desire to eat, and you may no longer take pleasure in eating. Treatment of your anxiety and/or your depression may result in regaining your lost weight.

Increased Physical Activity. If you have a high amplitude, marked tremor of both hands that is present most of the time, it may cause you to lose weight. The typical resting tremor that affects only one hand and is not constantly present does not result in weight loss. Likewise, if you develop marked dyskinesias while on levodopa/carbidopa, you will lose weight. Generally, you will only break down body fat and eventually your weight will stabilize.

Hypothalamus Malfunction. The hypothalamus sits above the pituitary gland, in front of the thalamus, and in the center of your ANS. The hypothalamus regulates your appetite by coordinating the actions of three hormones. One hormone is secreted by the stomach before you eat and increases your appetite, another is secreted by your fat cells and tells you that you're full, and the third is secreted by the hypothalamus and both increases food intake and decreases physical activity. The hypothalamus is affected in PD and it is theorized (but not proven) that the hypothalamus is "reset," so that you burn more calories than you take in, and thus lose weight.

Difficulty Swallowing. Significant difficulty swallowing, enough to cause you to lose weight, occurs late in PD. Symptoms of difficulty swallowing include taking longer to eat, coughing or choking while you eat, and drooling. If you have significant difficulty swallowing, you'll take longer to eat, you'll feel full and you'll eat less. If it's thought that your weight loss is related to difficulty swallowing and the loss is significant, you may require a feeding tube. However, in my experience it is rare for a patient to need a feeding tube due to weight loss from difficulty swallowing.

If you have lost a significant amount of weight you should be evaluated by your doctor.

38. Why do I sweat so much?

Sweat glands, called apocrine glands, release their secretions into hair follicles in your armpits, around your nipples, and in your groin. They're tubular glands that extend below the superficial layer of your skin into the deeper layer and produce a thick, cloudy secretion.

Sweat glands called **merocrine glands** are more numerous and widely distributed than apocrine glands and are more relevant in PD. Your skin contains almost three million merocrine glands. Your palms and soles have the highest number of them: 3,000 glands per square inch. Merocrine glands discharge their secretion, sweat, directly on your skin's surface. Sweat is 99% water, but it contains some salt. Merocrine glands have the following functions:

They cool your skin and reduce your body temperature. When all of your merocrine glands are working maximally, your rate of perspiration may exceed a gallon per hour, and fluid and salt losses can occur. For this reason, athletes in endurance sports must pause frequently to drink fluids.

Sweat glands

Tubular glands that are found nearly everywhere in the skin of humans and that secrete perspiration externally through pores to help regulate body temperature.

Merocrine glands

Sweat glands that discharge their secretion, sweat, directly on your skin's surface.

When all of your merocrine glands are working maximally, your rate of perspiration may exceed a gallon per hour, and fluid and salt losses can occur.

They provide protection from environmental hazards by diluting harmful chemicals and discouraging growth of bacteria.

In PD, increased sweating from merocrine glands may be the result of a malfunctioning ANS, and this may be complicated by anti-Parkinson drugs, especially levodopa/carbidopa. This is more likely to occur if you're on a high dose of levodopa/carbidopa and are experiencing "wearing off" and dyskinesia. In some patients the sweating is dramatic, with a patient having to change clothes several times a day or bedding several times a night. Such patients must be watched carefully and taught to keep up with loss of water and salt.

Sweating may become a problem, although some patients choose not to do anything, because sweating serves a purpose. Other patients apply an antiperspirant, 15% aluminum chloride hexahydrate—obtainable by prescription. The problem is that an antiperspirant applied to the arm pits and groin blocks sweating from apocrine, not merocrine glands (the main source of sweating). Similarly, Botox injections into the arm pits and groin only block secretions from apocrine glands. Nonetheless, in some patients this makes a difference. Finally, some patients use a beta-blocker, such as Inderal, that "turns down" the activity of the ANS. Care must be taken because patients who sweat excessively usually have orthostatic hypotension and a beta blocker can aggravate this.

At the Muhammad Ali Parkinson Center, we evaluate each patient who sweats profusely by making certain they don't have an overactive thyroid gland, diabetes, or are not going through menopause. We then devise a treatment plan that controls the sweating without causing additional problems.

PART FOUR

The First Five Years After You're Diagnosed

What is the goal of treatment?

What is a dopamine agonist?

I have Parkinson disease—why me?

As a care-partner, how can I cope with my partner's
Parkinson disease?

More . . .

39. What is the goal of treatment?

The goal of treatment is to provide you with the best possible quality of life. To do this, you must learn as much as you can about PD, work with your doctor, be willing to change your life—and you must have faith.

The goal of treatment is to provide you with the best possible quality of life. To do this, you must learn as much as you can about PD, work with your doctor, be willing to change your life—and you must have faith. In 40 years, I've evaluated 40,000 PD patients; I've seen what works and what doesn't and I've learned to be open-minded. Sometimes, today's "ridiculous ideas" are tomorrow's "wonder drugs." In 1944, when I was six, I had polio and was paralyzed from the waist down. The experts said I'd never walk again. As a child, I didn't believe it: I *did* walk—I was right and the experts were wrong.

Sometimes belief, faith, and a child's optimism trump science. As an expert, a neurologist, if I'd examined myself as a child, I too might have said I'd never walk again. Thank God for faith! Having learned to walk, although not perfectly, I graduated college and medical school, completed a rigorous and demanding internship, completed an even more rigorous and demanding neurology residency at Bellevue Hospital in New York, served in the United States Air Force, and became a professor—an "expert." Then, 15 years ago, the "impossible" happened and the polio came back as post-polio syndrome: a slow, relentless return of the weakness and paralysis I'd experienced 49 years earlier.

If you think defeating thoughts, you will be lost. Confront the "beast," whether it is PD or post-polio syndrome, and learn as much as you can about it. Do not despair and never stop trying. I find comfort from the Scriptures; you may find comfort from your own faith.

40. I move slowly and sometimes get stuck— are there exercises I can do?

In most patients, PD starts asymmetrically: on one side before the other. The asymmetry can appear as a lack of arm swing on one side, a turning-in or out of one foot, or a shuffling or scuffing of one foot. Our feet normally work as a team, so that if one foot slows down, as it does in PD, in time it forces the other foot to slow down as well. The exercises we emphasize at the Muhammad Ali Parkinson Clinic are ones that force both sides of your body to work together as a team in order to re-establish symmetry. We teach the following:

Walk with your spouse in front of you. She holds the front end of a walking stick in each of her hands, while you hold the back end of the walking sticks in each of yours. The walking sticks link you together like a bicycle built for two. She starts walking, swinging her arms and the walking sticks. This forces you to swing both your arms and to keep pace with her. Your arms and your legs are now working as a team.

Get on your hands and knees. Don't try this if you've had a knee and/or a hip replacement. Lower yourself to the floor on both hands and knees, then "walk" on your hands and knees. "Walking" this way forces you to move both your hands and feet symmetrically. A variant of this is to "walk" backwards on your hands and feet—this "re-programs" the sensors in your feet, as they're programmed to walk forward, not backward. This especially helps if you're having difficulty with balance or if you're "freezing." If you're walking on your hands and feet you can't fall and injure yourself. Another variant is to crawl, "commando-style," using your arms and legs to propel you forward. This also forces you to move both your hands and feet symmetrically.

Ride a stationary bicycle. Place a television set on a shelf in front of you, slightly above eye level. This forces you to look up at the television. This, in turn, forces your shoulder blades up and straightens out your spine. Now pedal—you're moving your arms and legs—symmetrically and in tandem.

Dance with your spouse. When you dance, you hold your partner, one arm around her waist, forcing your pelvis upward, and straightening your spine. The other arm is around her neck, forcing your shoulder blades upward, and also straightening your spine. The music, the rhythm, "takes over," and you move your arms and legs, rhythmically, symmetrically. Almost every PD patient will tell you they can dance much better than they can walk.

Swim. Some PD patients have difficulty swimming, they don't move an arm or a leg, and they "tip" to the side if they're not moving. When you swim, make sure someone is in the pool with you. Swim the breast stroke—it forces you to keep your eye on each arm, forcing you to move both arms, it forces your shoulder blades up, straightening your spine, and it tones and stretches your intercostal muscles, helping you breathe better.

Almost every PD patient will tell you they can dance much better than they can walk.

41. What about alternative drugs?

Alternative or complementary drugs and vitamins are non-prescription, off-patent, and have not been subjected to the vigorous trials prescription drugs undergo. For a prescription drug to be prescribed for PD, it must undergo extensive testing that follows these rules:

- The test must be *double-blind:* both the patient and investigator not knowing what drug the patient is on.
- The test must be *placebo-controlled:* the response of the patient to the drug compared to his response on the placebo.
- The test must be *multi-centered:* more than one medical center must test the drug to eliminate individual bias.

However, there are several alternative drugs that patients with PD use. There are drugs and foods that supplement levodopa, including **fava** or **broad beans**, which are widely eaten in the Mediterranean basin, including Spain, Italy, Greece, Turkey, Israel and the Middle East. They're an excellent source of fiber and have a high levodopa content; 3.5 ounces of fava beans are equivalent to 100 grams of levodopa if you're also taking carbidopa. If you're not taking carbidopa, 3.5 ounces of fava beans are the equivalent of 20 grams of levodopa. Warning: If you've never eaten fava beans, note that a small number of people may develop **anemia**, a disorder in which your red blood cells break down. If you're on a class of drugs called MAO-A inhibitors, or if you're on rasagiline or selegiline, you shouldn't eat fava beans.

Mucuna pruriens, or velvet beans, are widely eaten in India and Central America. Mucuna pruriens have a high protein and high levodopa content; 3.5 ounces of mucuna pruriens are equivalent to 100 grams of levodopa if you're taking carbidopa or 20 grams of levodopa if you're not. Touching the plant, but not the bean, causes itching—hence the name pruriens, or itching. It's been suggested, but not proven, that fava beans and mucuna pruriens are better sources of levodopa than levodopa/carbidopa pills. Many patients regularly eat

Fava

Fava is Italian for bean and refers specifically to the broad bean. Fava beans are the main commercial source of the drug L-DOPA.

Anemia

Low red blood cell counts that result in fatigue and dizziness.

fava beans and/or velvet beans (mucuna pruriens) and are convinced of their efficacy. I personally find them no different from levodopa/carbidopa pills.

The mitochondria in your cells require all the B vitamins for optimal functioning. How much of the B vitamins do your mitochondria need? We know your minimal daily requirement, the amount you need to prevent certain deficiency states, but this amount may not be the amount you need for optimal function. I recommend all my patients take at least one B-100 per day. This vitamin contains at least 100 mg of each of the B vitamins and a sufficient combination of niacin, folic acid and cyanocobalamine to decrease homocysteine levels. Homocysteine, an amino acid generated by levodopa/carbidopa, may be a risk factor for heart disease and stroke. As 100 mg of pyridoxine may interfere with the absorption of levodopa/carbidopa, I recommend taking the B-100 at least 4 hours before you take a dose of levodopa/carbidopa.

Coenzyme Q 10 is a carrier that transports charged particles from one complex to another in the mitochondria. As discussed in Question 31, it is also an antioxidant. It's not known how much Coenzyme Q 10 your mitochondria need. It is known that drugs that lower cholesterol (statins) also lower Coenzyme Q 10 levels. Some doctors tell their patients on statins to take Coenzyme Q 10. There is evidence that high doses of Coenzyme Q 10 *may* slow the progression of PD. At present, the National Institutes of Health (NIH) is conducting a study looking at the ability of 2,400 mg per day of Coenzyme Q 10 to slow the progression of PD. At present, without benefit of the NIH study, I do not recommend taking high doses of

Coenzyme Q 10. The efficacy is unproven and it is expensive.

Another category of alternative drugs is free radical scavengers (antioxidants) and metal chelators. Free radicals are charged particles that are able to attack and break down various components of the cell, especially the fat lining the cell and its organelles, the cell's RNA and DNA, and the cell's proteins: its vital enzymes, receptors, and transporters. Antioxidants can be water soluble, like vitamin C, or fat soluble, like vitamin E. As discussed in Question 31, it is unclear if antioxidants penetrate the cell in sufficient quantities to be effective. Some free radical scavengers/antioxidants such as alpha lipoic acid, gluthathione, and N acetyl cysteine have already been mentioned. Additional free radical scavengers include:

Curcumin, the active substance in curry powder, is an antioxidant and an anti-inflammatory drug. Some experts attribute the relative low prevalence of Alzheimer's disease in India to the wide-spread use of curry. **Ginseng**, the dried root of an herb, is also an antioxidant. There are several ginseng preparations and different claims are made for each. However, at present there is insufficient information to recommend either curcumin or ginseng.

Green tea contains a number of chemicals called polyphenols that are antioxidants. Several of these polyphenols are being studied for their ability to halt the progression of PD and Alzheimer's disease. Drinking 4 to 8 cups of green tea is not unreasonable. If you enjoy green tea—drink it, it's probably good for you.

Ginseng

A herb that has been used to stimulate the adrenal gland and thereby increase energy. It also may have some beneficial effect on reducing blood sugar in patients with diabetes mellitus.

Green tea

Tea made from leaves that are not fermented before being dried.

Acetylcholine

A chemical that acts to transmit nerve impulses in the brain, the peripheral nerves, the heart, the gut, the bladder, and the muscles.

Acetylcholine, a chemical messenger, is decreased in the brains of people with Alzheimer's disease and Lewy Body Disease (LBD). Acetylcholine is also a chemical messenger in the gut, bladder, and testes. Increased acetylcholine levels are said to improve memory, combat apathy, decrease anxiety and depression, combat fatigue, increase energy, aid digestion and constipation, and to combat impotence. These claims were not generated by double-blind, placebo-controlled, multi-center studies and must be viewed skeptically. And with some of the drugs it's unclear if they actually increase acetylcholine levels in the brain and other tissues. Among the acetylcholine "enhancers" that people take are: Acetyl L-carnitine, curcumin, cytidine-5-diphosphocholine, ginseng, and licorice.

Other alternative drugs include:

St. John's Wort, an herb, increases brain serotonin levels. Serotonin is a chemical messenger involved in regulating behavior, mood, and sleep. St. John's Wort has been found to be effective in treating some forms of depression, though I've not found it effective in treating the depression of PD. In some people, St. John's Wort may increase bleeding.

Magnesium chloride is a muscle relaxant used to treat pre-eclampsia (high blood pressure associated with pregnancy), as well as anxiety, chorea, and muscle spasms. I've not found it helpful in treating levodopa-induced dyskinesias nor in treating dystonic muscle spasms.

Melatonin is a hormone secreted by the pineal gland. At a dose of one to three milligrams, melatonin increases brain levels of serotonin, a chemical messenger that regulates sleep, though I've occasionally found it helpful in treating the sleep disorder of PD.

42. What is a dopamine agonist?

A dopamine *antagonist* is a drug, such as Compazine, Haldol, or Thorazine, that blocks dopamine receptors in the brain. These drugs cause a form of Parkinson disease that is reversible when the drug is stopped. A **dopamine agonist** is the opposite of an antagonist. Agonists, like dopamine itself, excite or stimulate dopamine receptors in the brain. Unlike levodopa, agonists work directly and do not have to be changed to dopamine by a decreasing number of inefficient neurons in the substantia nigra.

There are at least five types of dopamine receptors in the brain: D-1, D-2, D-3, D-4, and D-5. The D-1 and D-2 receptors are located on neurons in the putamen, and are the targets of the neurons in the substantia nigra. The D-1 and D-2 neurons are important in PD. The D-3, D-4, and D-5 receptors are on neurons in other regions of the brain: the mesolimbic and mesocortical regions. These neurons may be important in regulating anxiety, depression, and compulsive behavior. Dopamine formed from levodopa stimulates both the D-1 and the D-2 receptors, which is why it is so effective. But this may also be why levodopa causes dyskinesias. The dopamine agonists stimulate a different combination of receptors. Mirapex (pramipexole) and Requip (ropinirole) stimulate the D-2, D-3, and D-4 receptors. They tend to be less effective than Sinemet, but don't cause dyskinesia. Mirapex also has an anti-depressant effect in some people. Unfortunately, because they stimulate the neurons regulating compulsive behavior, Mirapex, Requip, and **Neupro** (rotigotine) may cause compulsive eating, gambling,

Dopamine agonist
Drug that exerts its pharmacologic effects by directly activating dopamine agonist receptors.

Agonists, like dopamine itself, excite or stimulate dopamine receptors in the brain.

Neupro
Neupro (rotigotine) is used to treat early signs and symptoms of Parkinson's disease.

shopping, or sexual behavior in a small number of patients (perhaps 5%).

The agonists Mirapex, Requip, and Neupro have been shown through clinical research to be so effective in treating people with early PD that the need for levodopa/carbidopa may be delayed for several years. There is less risk of developing wearing off, "on-off," dystonia, and dyskinesias with the agonists than with levodopa/carbidopa. This is primarily due to the short half-life of levodopa, which is approximately 90 minutes. A half-life of 90 minutes means that after that time, the peak dose level of the drug has decreased by half (or 50%). After another 90 minutes the dose level will have decreased by another 50%. Most drugs are eliminated from the body and their effectiveness is gone, after five half-lives. The half-life gives you an idea as to how frequently you must take a drug to maintain effective circulating levels of the drug. However, drugs that enter the brain (such as levodopa and the dopamine agonists) are stored there and may continue to be active even after they have been eliminated from the body on the basis of their half-lives.

The short half-life of levodopa results in alternating high and low blood and brain levels of, first levodopa, then dopamine. It's this alternation of high and low levels of dopamine that's thought to lead to wearing-off, dystonia, and dyskinesia. It's as though you keep hitting the dopamine receptors with a "jack-hammer" until you finally change their sensitivity. Dopamine agonists have a much longer half-life, thus prolonging the stimulation of the receptors and delaying the development of wearing-off, dystonia, and dyskinesia.

Mirapex, one of the dopamine agonists, is usually started at a dose of 0.25 mg three times a day. Talk to your doctor about what dose will be most effective for you. The half-life of Mirapex is 8 hours, so if you take doses too closely together you're more likely to have side effects: drowsiness, dizziness on standing (orthostatic hypotension), and nausea. Discuss any side effects you have with your doctor. In some patients, Mirapex has a specific anti-tremor effect. I led a large, multicentered, double-blind, placebo-controlled study of patients with advanced PD that showed Mirapex, at a mean dose of 3.0 mg per day, could lower the dose of levodopa/carbidopa by almost two tablets (200 mg of levodopa) while maintaining a comparable anti-Parkinson effect, increasing the number of hours patients were "on" or mobile, and decreasing the prevalence and severity of dyskinesias. The study was published in *Neurology* in 1997.

Another dopamine agonist, Requip, is also usually started at a dose of 0.25 mg three times a day. Side effects may be similar to those of Mirapex. Again, discuss proper dosing and side effects with your doctor. A new preparation of Requip, Requip-XL (Requip extended release) has recently become available. Requip XL is administered once a day and appears more helpful. On a mg per mg basis, Requip XL is at least as effective as regular Requip in patients with early, newly diagnosed PD, as well as those with advanced PD. Patients can easily be switched from regular Requip to Requip XL.

Mirapex's main route of elimination is the kidneys, while Requip's main route of elimination is the liver. Drugs like Mirapex that are eliminated through the kidney are less likely to lead to drug-drug interactions. Drug-drug interactions are always a consideration in older patients who are on multiple drugs for disorders other than PD, such as heart disease, hypertension, hypercholesterolemia, diabetes, and overactive bladder. Drugs like Requip, which are eliminated through the liver, are more likely to have a larger "spread" in their dosing level. In patients who will be treated for several years, the availability of a larger dosing spread is invaluable in managing them.

Neupro, or rotigotine, can be characterized as a dopamine receptor agonist with a preference for the D3 receptor over D2 and D1 receptors. In addition, it exhibits interaction with D4 and D5 receptors, the role of the D4 and D5 receptors is, as yet, unclear in PD. Neupro is fat soluble, which allows it to be administered through a patch applied to the skin. The patch, applied once per day, releases rotigotine at a constant rate over 24 hours. The drug bypasses the gut and is metabolized in the liver. The patch has been shown to be effective in newly diagnosed patients with early PD, as well as in patients with advanced PD who are already on levodopa/carbidopa. The Neupro patch increases the amount of time spent in "on" or mobile periods, and decreases the prevalence of dyskinesias.

Table 4 shows equivalent doses of levodopa/carbidopa, Mirapex, Requip, Requip XL, and Neupro.

43. What are the side effects of dopamine agonists?

One of the side effects people experience when taking dopamine agonists is **drowsiness**. Periods of daytime drowsiness, sometimes accompanied by falling asleep, occur in people with PD who are not on any treatment, those with PD who are taking levodopa/carbidopa, and those on an agonist. The periods of drowsiness, which may be more frequent for those taking an agonist,

Drowsiness

A state of impaired awareness associated with a desire or inclination to sleep.

Table 4   Equivalent Doses

Drug	Equivalent dose to 100 mg of levodopa/carbidopa
Levodopa/carbidopa	100 mg
Mirapex	1.0 mg
Requip	3.0 mg
Requip XL	3.0 mg
Neupro	2.0 mg

may be embarrassing (if you fall asleep while a friend is talking to you), and may even be dangerous if you fall asleep while driving. If you experience daytime drowsiness, do not drive until you've talked to your doctor. The periods of drowsiness usually disappear. If you experience drowsiness on Mirapex or Requip, talk to your doctor about how to pace your doses. Sometimes I prescribe a drug, such as Pro-vigil, that promotes alertness.

If you experience nausea, talk to your doctor about reducing your starting dose.

Nausea may occur if you're started on Mirapex, Requip, Requip XL, or levodopa/carbidopa as your first anti-Parkinson drug. Drugs that stimulate dopamine receptors in your basal ganglia also stimulate dopamine receptors in your gut and in a region of your brain called the medulla, which contains the "vomiting center." It may take several days or weeks for your body to successfully accommodate the first anti-Parkinson drugs your doctor prescribes. If you experience nausea, talk to your doctor about reducing your starting dose. If nausea persists, I often prescribe Tigan, an **antihistamine**, to be taken one hour before each dose of

Antihistamine

A medicine used to treat allergies and hypersensitive reactions and colds; works by counteracting the effects of histamine on a receptor site.

125

Mirapex or Requip. After a month, Tigan is usually not needed. For nausea unresponsive to Tigan, I prescribe domperidone (Motilium), a drug available from Canada. Domperidone specifically blocks dopamine receptors in the gut and vomiting center, but not in the basal ganglia (where it would aggravate PD). Do not use drugs such as Compazine or Reglan: these drugs successfully block dopamine receptors in the gut and vomiting center, but also block dopamine receptors in the basal ganglia and can worsen PD.

By starting with a low dose of an agonist, you are not as likely to experience as quick and as dramatic an improvement as on levodopa/carbidopa. But by starting low, and going slowly, substantial improvement will occur within several weeks and you will maintain it longer. The management of nausea associated with levodopa/carbidopa is discussed later.

Dizziness or *lightheadedness* on standing, another possible side effect, usually indicates a drop in blood pressure called postural or orthostatic hypotension. Postural or orthostatic hypotension may occur because you are dehydrated, diabetic, taking drugs to lower your blood pressure, taking a diuretic (a "water" pill), or because you have PD. If you experience dizziness on standing when you start an agonist, try sitting on the edge of your bed for a few minutes before standing up, or try not taking your blood pressure drugs at the same time that you take your agonist, or try lying down for an hour after you take your agonist. After one or two weeks most people are able to tolerate the agonist. If dizziness on standing persists, your doctor may consider starting you on a different agonist, a different anti-Parkinson drug, or adding a drug that counter-acts your postural hypotension.

Edema, or swelling of the legs, occurs in less than 5% of people on an agonist. It's usually mild and responds to lowering the dose of the agonist. Rarely, the agonist must be stopped. The edema does not usually respond to diuretics (water pills). Some doctors are unaware of the potential of agonists to cause edema, and your doctor may be concerned that you are experiencing heart failure or that you have a blood clot in a leg vein (phlebitis). If neither of these situations is accurate, then the edema is likely related to the agonist. If edema occurs on Mirapex, it may also occur on Requip or on Neupro, though there are so many exceptions to the rule that if you experience edema while on one of the agonists, it's worth trying a different one.

Edema
Swelling of the legs.

A small number of PD patients, perhaps 2% to 5%, develop *compulsive* or *driven* or *disinhibited behavior*. The behavior may consist of compulsive eating (characterized by a craving for chocolates and sweets), compulsive shopping (going on "sprees" and buying unnecessary goods and services), compulsive gambling (gambling in casinos, on the internet, playing the lottery), and compulsive sexual behavior (viewing pornography, soliciting phone sex or prostitutes). Because of their dramatic nature, compulsive gambling and compulsive sexual behavior have received a disproportionate amount of press coverage and notoriety. Compulsive behavior occurs in some PD patients not on any drugs, in some patients on levodopa/carbidopa, after deep brain stimulation, as well as in some patients on dopamine agonists. If you're on a dopamine agonist you should be told of the small possibility that it may cause compulsive behavior and that if you experience strong drives or urges you must talk to your doctor. Often reducing the dose of the agonist or levodopa/carbidopa is enough to control the behavior.

A small number of PD patients, perhaps 2% to 5%, develop compulsive or driven or disinhibited behavior.

Sometimes you have to change agonists, and sometimes you have to stop them altogether. The "harm" comes from not knowing the compulsive behavior may be drug-related.

Hallucinations

A delusion in which a person sees or hears things or people that don't exist.

Delusion

A belief in something with no basis in reality.

Some patients, especially patients 75 years or older, may have **hallucinations**, **delusions**, or confusion on levodopa/carbidopa as well as on dopamine agonists, amantadine or tri-hexiphenidyl (Artane). The hallucinations are usually visual: seeing things, animals, or people that aren't there. You may or may not realize these hallucinations are not real. Some hallucinations can be benign, or even pleasant, while some are frightening and may be accompanied by agitation, anxiety, and panic. Agonists are more likely than levodopa/carbidopa to cause hallucinations because they are longer acting.

Hallucinations are more likely to occur in older people because they're more likely to be developing a dementia. Treatment of the hallucinations consists of understanding why you're having them. If you have an infection, are dehydrated, or if you're in a strange place, you may have hallucinations. If the hallucinations are related to your anti-Parkinson drug, reducing or stopping the drug usually aborts the hallucinations. Hallucinations result from stimulation of specific regions of the brain that contain receptors for the chemical serotonin. These serotonin receptors are stimulated by the hallucination-generating drug LSD. A new class of drugs, exemplified by pimavanserin, blocks the serotonin receptors, and blocks hallucinations. Currently, pimavanserin is an experimental drug, one that is still undergoing testing.

Delusions are beliefs that aren't real. You may believe your spouse or care-partner is trying to hurt you, steal from you, poison you, or have you put away. Such delusions are called **paranoia**. These delusions may be accompanied by hallucinations. If the delusions are related to your anti-Parkinson drugs, reducing or stopping the drug usually stops the delusions. Sometimes a drug, called a neuroleptic, is prescribed to counteract the delusions. Unfortunately, the neuroleptic drugs may also aggravate the symptoms of Parkinson disease. The serotonin-blocking drug, pimavanserin, blocks delusions without aggravating Parkinson disease.

Paranoia

A belief that people are seeking to harm you.

44. What is an MAO-B inhibitor?

Monoamine oxidase (MAO) is an enzyme found in mitochondria that exists in two forms: MAO-A and MAO-B. MAO-A breaks down adrenalin, noradrenalin, and serotonin, and is found predominantly in cells lining the gut, liver, and in neurons of the brain. MAO-B breaks down dopamine and is found in the brain, primarily in the neurons of the substantia nigra. Drugs that block MAO-A, called MAO-A inhibitors are used to treat severe depression. Drugs that inhibit MAO-B increase dopamine in the brain and improve the symptoms of PD.

Selegiline (Eldepryl) was the first MAO-B inhibitor approved for use in PD. In a study conducted by Drs. Golbe, Muenter, and myself, selegiline (10mg/day) was shown to decrease "wearing off" in patients taking levodopa. Zelapar is a form of selegiline that dissolves on the tongue and is rapidly absorbed in the blood stream. Zelapar bypasses the stomach, intestines, and liver, and thus reaches the brain more rapidly. Because it increases and prolongs the effects of levodopa (either the levodopa normally formed in the neurons or the levodopa that is formed from carbidopa/levodopa), Zelapar decreases the "wearing off" that occurs in all patients after they've been on levodopa for several months or years.

Rasagiline (Azilect)

Rasagiline (trade name Azilect) is an irreversible inhibitor of monoamine oxidase used as a monotherapy in early Parkinson's disease.

Rasagiline (Azilect) is another MAO-B inhibitor, developed by Dr. Moussa Youdim, a developer of selegiline. A clinical study by the Parkinson Study Group showed rasagiline to be effective in treating PD patients' symptoms. Rasagiline can also be used as an adjunct to levodopa in patients with advanced PD and, like Zelapar, has shown to be effective in decreasing the wearing off of levodopa. A recent study suggests that rasagiline, started early, may delay the appearance of some of the symptoms of Parkinson disease. Additional studies are in progress to determine if rasagiline may delay the progression of Parkinson disease.

Rasagiline and selegiline used alone tend to delay the appearance of freezing of gait (FOG), a troublesome symptom of advanced PD. In patients who are already experiencing FOG the addition of these medications may reduce the FOG effects. Patients taking MAO-B inhibitors are cautioned about the interaction of these drugs with over-the-counter cold preparations, diet pills, and narcotic pain relief (such as Demerol). It is best to consult with your doctor regarding possible side effects.

In 1961, Walter Birkmayer was the first doctor to administer levodopa to PD patients. He subsequently reported, in 1986 (in the *Journal of Neural Transmission*), on a retrospective study of 941 patients he'd treated over 10 years. He reported that patients on deprenyl (selegiline) and levodopa lived longer than patients on levodopa alone. He postulated that selegiline had a neuroprotective effect: that it delayed the progression of PD. Subsequent studies showed that selegiline, given before MPTP, a toxin that causes a

Parkinson-like disorder, blocked the development of PD in monkeys. These observations led, in 1987, to the DATATOP study, Deprenyl (selegiline) and Tocopherol (vitamin E) Antioxidative Therapy of Parkinsonism. After 14 months of controlled observation, 10 mg of selegiline per day was found to significantly delay the time when enough disability developed to warrant the initiation of levodopa. The effect was sustained during the overall 8.2 years of observation. Most experts have interpreted the DATATOP study as showing that selegiline delays the time until levodopa is needed because selegiline itself has an anti-Parkinson effect. Some experts interpret DATATOP as suggesting selegiline is neuroprotective. Some experts also interpret a recent study, called ADAGIO, as suggesting that rasagiline may also be neuroprotective: that it may delay the progression of Parkinson disease.

45. What is Amantadine?

Amantadine may improve PD by releasing dopamine from the neurons in the substantia nigra, or by blocking the production of acetylcholine. Drugs that block acetylcholine increase the activity of dopamine. Side effects of amantadine include a reddish-violet discoloration of the legs called "livedo reticularis." This may be accompanied by swelling, but the discoloration and swelling disappear when amantadine is stopped. In older people (age 70 plus) amantadine may cause hallucinations, but again, the hallucinations stop when amantadine is stopped.

It has been found that amantadine decreases levodopa-induced dyskinesia. The effect on dyskinesia is related to amantadine's ability to block a type of receptor called an NMDA receptor, a receptor for the amino acid glutamate. Glutamate is involved in exciting, rather than inhibiting, blocking, or depressing nerve cells. However, too much glutamate, like too much excitement, isn't good. NMDA receptors hook onto glutamate and let it do its work of exciting the cell, but these NMDA receptors may become overly sensitive, which results in dyskinesia. By blocking the NMDA receptors, amantadine decreases dyskinesia.

46. What are anticholinergic drugs?

Anticholinergic drugs, such as Artane and Cogentin, block the actions of acetylcholine. Normally acetylcholine slows your heart, constricts your pupils, contracts your bladder, and increases salivation, gut motility, and sweating. Blocking acetylcholine in the periphery (outside the brain) can have both good and bad effects. The good effects include stopping you from drooling and relaxing an overactive bladder. The bad effects include increased heart rate, constipation, and blurred vision.

Central brain effects of anticholinergic drugs relieve tremor. In the basal ganglia, acetylcholine acts as a chemical neurotransmitter and can function as a "brake" on dopamine. Anticholinergic drugs decrease acetylcholine and in effect "increase" dopamine. Side effects of anticholinergic drugs include dry mouth, constipation, urinary retention, confusion, disorientation, memory loss, and hallucinations. Older patients (70 and over) are more susceptible to these side effects.

47. Why am I feeling anxious?

Your body's reaction to anxiety is controlled by your autonomic nervous system (ANS), which, when you are anxious, can be "tricked" into making your heart beat faster, making you feel dizzy or lightheaded, or making you breathe faster so that you hyperventilate.

Anxiety or stress is a mixture of fear, uncertainty, and worry. In the right proportion, these feelings are survival skills. Our ancestors, living in a primitive society, would not have survived if they weren't anxious, uncertain, and fearful, didn't suspect danger around every rock, behind every tree, inside every cave. If our ancestors didn't worry, weren't fearful about being pounced upon by a hungry lion, or getting back to their cave before dark, they wouldn't have survived. However, anxiety, stress, fear, uncertainty, and worry in the absence of real danger aren't survival traits, they're bad for you: they prematurely age you and every organ in your body, including your brain.

Anxiety or stress is a mixture of fear, uncertainty, and worry. In the right proportion, these feelings are survival skills.

Anxiety, fear, uncertainty, and worry are everywhere and at different times we use different words to convey these feelings. Words commonly used include: afraid, irritable, nervous, stressed, tense, terrified, panicked. Each conveys a different shade of meaning, but it's the same idea, the same feeling: one of anticipation, or uncertainty. Often, stress and anxiety are expressed not in words but in physical symptoms, which are commonly: feeling dizzy, flushed, faint, unsteady, or wobbly. Unrecognized and untreated stress is an aggravating factor in most diseases including Parkinson disease. And stress shortens life. People who live longer do not necessarily have less stress, rather they've learned to cope with and manage their stress.

The question is not whether you're stressed; we all are to some extent. The question is whether the stress is proportionate or disproportionate to what you're doing or going through. Another important question is how the stress is impacting your life. To better understand stress and anxiety, you can measure it the way you measure fever or blood pressure. A guide for doing this is the Anxiety Scale (**Table 5**).

Table 5 Anxiety Scale

For the past week, rate the following symptoms on a scale of:
0 = symptom absent; 1 = symptom mild; 2 = symptom moderate;
3 = symptom moderate to marked; 4 = symptom marked to severe,
incapacitating

 1 Do you feel anxious?
 2 Do you feel afraid or fearful?
 3 Do you feel uncertain?
 4 Do you feel worried?
 5 Do you feel nervous or irritable?

 6 Do you feel you can't concentrate or pay attention?
 7 Do you feel insecure, like you're losing control?
 8 Do you feel terrified?
 9 Do you feel stressed or tense?
10 Do you feel panicked?

11 Do you feel your hands or feet tingling or burning?
12 Do you feel flushed? Have hot or cold flashes? Feel like you're sweating?
13 Do you feel dizzy or light-headed?
14 Do you feel faint?
15 Do you easily fatigue or tire?

16 Do you feel your vision's blurred? Or your ears are ringing?
17 Do you feel like you're choking?
18 Do you feel your heart pounding? Do you feel pressure on your chest?
19 Do you feel short of breath?
20 Do you feel nauseated? Or feel like vomiting?

21 Do you feel a frequent urge to urinate or move your bowels?
22 Do you feel you can't fall asleep, or stay asleep?
23 Do you feel unsteady, or wobbly, or off balance?
24 Do you feel your hands or feet shaking or trembling?
25 Do you feel restless, or jumpy?

0–6:	No Anxiety
7–11:	Mild Anxiety
12–25:	Moderate-Marked Anxiety

Part of learning to calm yourself is to learn to listen to your internal organs and then learn to control them. For example, if your stomach aches or your bowels are distended, they may be reacting to stress. If your lungs are over-breathing and you are dizzy or light-headed, your lungs may be telling you that you are stressed. Likewise if your heart pounds or races, it too may be telling you that you are stressed. Managing the stress of day-to-day living is a key to living better with PD. In any group of PD patients at least 50% will, at some time during the course of their PD, be moderately to markedly stressed, enough to consult a psychologist or psychiatrist, to seek counseling for managing stress, or use a prescription drug to manage their stress. Along with those options there are several techniques you can use to calm yourself.

Meditation. Meditation consists of focusing your mind on a single calming image or thought and excluding all stressful images and thoughts. Meditation teaches you to "turn-on" your inner calming center. When you meditate, sit in a comfortable position and breathe in a calm, easy way. Quiet your mind, slow down your thoughts, and focus your attention on one thing. Some people chant while they meditate.

Faith. Practicing your faith through prayer or worship can calm you and provide a sense that you are not alone.

Repetitive exercises. These should be done daily for up to an hour each morning—before the stress of the day begins. And, if necessary, should be repeated for up to an hour in the evening if the day has been stressful. Repetitive exercises may include riding a stationary bicycle, running in place or on a treadmill, jogging, rowing, swimming laps, or walking.

Practicing your faith through prayer or worship can calm you and provide a sense that you are not alone.

48. Why do I have trouble falling asleep?

Approximately 50% of all people with PD have difficulty sleeping at night. In some it is a minor nuisance, but for a few it is a major problem.

Temporary insomnia lasting less than 4 weeks is self-limited and has no serious repercussions. Temporary insomnia occurs in up to 50% of all people and is more frequent in older people, shift workers, international travelers, and people under stress. Chronic insomnia, such as occurs in PD, lasts longer than 4 weeks, is not self-limited, and may have repercussions. Such insomnia usually results in daytime fatigue, grogginess, irritability, mood swings, and difficulty paying attention or concentrating. People with chronic insomnia are more likely to suffer from anxiety, depression, mood swings, or paranoia. Whether these disorders came first and insomnia is part of them or whether the insomnia came first and unmasked them is a source of debate. In discussing insomnia with the doctor, be prepared to answer questions such as these:

What time do you go to bed?

How long does it take for you to fall asleep?

While trying to fall asleep, what do you do?

Do you wake up during the night? For what reason?

How many times do you wake up?

How many hours do you sleep?

When do usually wake up?

After you wake up, do you get up or stay in bed? How long?

When you wake up are you refreshed or groggy?

Do you nap during the day? More than once?

Your bed partner is a valuable source of information because most people are unaware of their behavior while sleeping. Your bed partner is probably the only one who can comment on specific behaviors: talking in your sleep, crying or shouting, snoring (which may indicate sleep apnea), thrashing or kicking, or walking in your sleep.

Preparing to answer questions such as those listed will help you and your doctor to identify the cause of your insomnia. Just telling your doctor that you can't sleep without first analyzing your sleep habits isn't helpful. Treatment consists of teaching you sleep hygiene including:

Going to bed only when you're sleepy, leaving the bedroom if you're unable to fall asleep within 30 minutes and returning to the bedroom only when you're sleepy, and waking up at the same time every morning, including weekends. Some insomniacs unwittingly engage in activities that aggravate the problem, including excessive use of stimulants such as coffee or caffeine-containing soft drinks, sleeping excessively on weekends, or daytime napping. Many insomniacs become preoccupied with their difficulty sleeping, and as worry and concern tend to peak around bedtime, this worsens the insomnia. There are additional reasons why people with PD have difficulty sleeping at night. Often, there is more than one reason a person has difficulty sleeping, and if this is so, all reasons must be addressed.

Difficulty Sleeping Related to PD. It's normal during sleep for people to awaken during the night—to roll over, change positions, and then to fall back asleep. PD patients may awaken and find themselves so rigid they're unable to change positions and can't go back to sleep. To turn over in bed requires you to first raise your arm over your head, then using your arm as

Your bed partner is probably the only one who can comment on specific behaviors: talking in your sleep, crying or shouting, snoring (which may indicate sleep apnea), thrashing or kicking, or walking in your sleep.

a "lever," to flip yourself over. An early symptom of PD is a decreased arm swing when walking. You may not realize that at night the decreased arm swing results in an inability to raise your arm and use it as a lever to flip yourself over. Simple instructions on how to turn in bed at night is occasionally the only sleep aid required. If difficulty turning or moving in bed at night is related to the timing of your last dose of levodopa, a short-acting drug, a dopamine agonist, or a long-acting drug may help.

Difficulty Sleeping Related to PD Drugs. Drugs that help you stay awake during the day can interfere with your sleep at night. Because you took the drug early in the day doesn't mean it has been cleared from your body and your brain. Drugs patients with PD use that might cause difficulty sleeping at night include:

- Selegiline (Eldepryl) keeps some patients awake at night because it is metabolized to amphetamine. If you're taking selegiline, consider not taking it after 12:00 noon.
- Modafinil (Pro-vigil) is used to treat daytime drowsiness by inhibiting the reuptake of norepinephrine in the locus ceruleus, a sleep center located near the substantia nigra.
- Diuretics ("water pills"), taken at night, will cause you to urinate frequently, which will keep you awake at night going to the bathroom.

Difficulty Sleeping Related to a Sleep Disorder. Sleep is NOT a passive process, the absence of being awake. Sleep is an active process, one necessary for the proper functioning of your brain. Sleep follows a regular cycle each night and consists of both slow wave sleep (SWS) and rapid eye movement (REM) sleep. The regions regulating sleep are in your brainstem, a region uniquely positioned to regulate sleep because it regulates eye opening and closing, eye movements, posture, and tone. The regions regulating sleep are near your substantia nigra, the region most affected in PD. The diagnosis of a primary sleep disorder is made in the absence of other causes of insomnia. One of the more common sleep disorders is obstructive sleep apnea.

Obstructive sleep apnea is a potentially life-threatening condition that's more common than generally appreciated. Sleep apnea is a breathing disorder characterized by brief interruptions of respirations during sleep. It's estimated that 18 million Americans, 6% of the population, may have sleep apnea. People likely to have sleep apnea include those who snore loudly, who are overweight, who have high blood pressure, or who have some physical abnormality of the nose, throat, or other parts of the upper airway. This includes people with PD. In some people, sleep apnea is inherited. The treatment of a primary sleep disorder may involve consultation with a sleep expert and a night spent in a sleep lab.

Commonly used nonprescription, over-the-counter drugs include melatonin, a hormone secreted by the pineal gland and thought to regulate circadian rhythms. Another drug is **diphenydramine** (Benadryl) an antihistamine. Benadryl may result in drowsiness without sleep. An added benefit is that Benadryl has an anti-tremor effect.

Commonly used prescription drugs include benzodiazepines, a class of drugs that bind to a special receptor in the brain, called the benzodiazepine receptor. Benzodiazepines include sedating drugs such as temazepam (Restoril), but also include non-sedating drugs such as clonazepam (Klonopin), alprazolam (Xanax), diazepam (Valium), and lorazepam (Ativan). Potential problems

Obstructive sleep apnea is a potentially life-threatening condition that's more common than generally appreciated. Sleep apnea is a breathing disorder characterized by brief interruptions of respirations during sleep.

Diphenydramine

Antihistamine (trade name Benadryl) used to treat allergic reactions involving the nasal passages (hay fever) and also to treat motion sickness.

139

with benzodiazepines include rapid accommodation (you get used to the drug in a few weeks), non-refreshing sleep, drowsiness on awakening, memory lapses, unsteadiness, and the risk of becoming addicted.

Your doctor may prescribe an antidepressant with sleep-inducing properties. Mirtazapine (Remeron) is a mild anti-depressant and has anti-tremor activity. Trazadone (Desyrel) is a tricyclic antidepressant with sedating properties and relatively few side effects. A new class of sleep-promoting drugs, drugs that increase the percent of REM sleep, include eszopiclone (Lunesta), zalepon (Sonata), zolpidem (Ambien), and ramelton (Rozerem).

49. What is restless legs syndrome (RLS)?

Restless Legs Syndrome (RLS) is an uncomfortable, aching sensation that's relieved by constantly moving your legs in bed or by walking. RLS implies that movement, restlessness, is part of the syndrome but it's not. RLS is a sensory disorder; the movement—the restlessness—is voluntary, an attempt by you to relieve the uncomfortable sensation. RLS occurs in 10%—15% of all people, and in about 10% of them the symptoms are sufficiently severe to consult a neurologist. RLS may be more common in PD, occurring in approximately 20% of patients. RLS may begin at any age, but most people are affected after age 50. About 80% of people with RLS experience periodic limb movements (PLM) during sleep.

People describe RLS as an irresistible urge to move in order to overcome a twitching, burning, aching sensation felt in the calf muscles. Some patients describe it as though your feet were plunged into ice water and kept there for several minutes. Occasionally, the sensation involves the feet or thighs, and rarely the arms or hands. Relief is obtained by getting up and walking, which can be difficult for someone with PD. Because RLS occurs at night and is relieved by walking around, it usually results in insomnia and daytime drowsiness. Diabetes, iron deficiency anemia, kidney disease, peripheral neuropathy, and poor circulation can all cause RLS. However, most of the time, the cause of RLS is not known. Dopamine agonists help RLS, while dopamine antagonists worsen RLS, suggesting dopamine plays a role in this syndrome. The dopamine agonists ropinirole (Requip) and pramipexole (Mirapex) have shown to be effective in treating RLS. If you think you have RLS, you may want to take the International RLS Questionnaire in **Table 6** or consult your doctor.

Diabetes, iron deficiency anemia, kidney disease, peripheral neuropathy, and poor circulation can all cause restless legs syndrome (RLS).

Periodic limb movements, as just mentioned, consist of kicking, thrashing, crying out, or shouting while asleep. PLM occurs during REM sleep and is associated with vivid and often frightening dreams. REM sleep disorders can result from levodopa and are best treated by reducing the dose of levodopa or by adding an atypical dopamine blocking drug such as quetiapine (Seroquel). Although 80% of people with PLM have RLS and RLS is treated with a dopamine agonist, the agonists do not aggravate PLM. This is because the dose of the agonist needed to treat RLS is not high enough to provoke PLM.

50. Can I still have sex if I have Parkinson disease?

PD drugs raise dopamine levels in the brain, including the hypothalamus, which stimulates the thyroid and adrenal glands as well as the testes and ovaries. Dopamine allows men and women to feel sexually

Table 6 International Restless Legs Questionnaire

For the past week, rate the following on a scale of: 0 = absent, none; 1 = mild; 2 = moderate; 3 = marked, severe; 4 = very severe, incapacitating

Score					Symptom
0	1	2	3	4	Rate the discomfort, the RLS, in your legs or arms
0	1	2	3	4	Rate the need to move because of your discomfort or RLS
0	1	2	3	4	How much relief of RLS do you get from moving?
0	1	2	3	4	How severely does RLS disturb your sleep?
0	1	2	3	4	How severely does RLS cause daytime tiredness or sleepiness?
0	1	2	3	4	Overall how severe is your RLS?
0	1 [1 day]	2 [2–3 days]	3 [3–5 days]	4 [6–7 days]	How many days per week do you get RLS?
0	1 [Less than one hour]	2 [1–3 hours]	3 [3–8 hours]	4 [8–24 hours]	When you have an episode of RLS, how long does it last?
0	1	2	3	4	How severe is the impact of RLS on your ability to carry out a satisfactory family, home, social, school, or work life?
0	1	2	3	4	How often does RLS result in your being angry, anxious, depressed, irritable, moody, or sad?

1–10 = mild RLS; 11–20 = moderate RLS; 21–30 = severe RLS; 31–40 = incapacitating RLS aroused, but other factors may interfere with performance and desire. These factors include erectile dysfunction, difficulty moving and turning in bed, inability to perform in a certain position, lack of estrogen or testosterone, anxiety, depression, paranoia, and adverse drug effects.

Forty percent of men and women with PD, and an almost equal number of aged people, lose interest in sex or are unable to have sex. Just how PD contributes to loss of desire and its impact on sexuality is not clear. It is not uncommon for sexual desires to decrease later in life, but because PD affects the autonomic nervous system, it may lessen the response to sexual stimulation. For women, menopause brings hormonal changes and some women experience a decreased desire for sexual relationships. However, a woman with PD may also feel that her symptoms have robbed her of her femininity and she may feel less attractive and less desirable as a sexual partner. For older men, sexual dysfunction or the inability to achieve or maintain an erection can affect their self-esteem.

Blood flow throughout the body must be sufficient for sexual organs to work satisfactorily. For example, during arousal, the human penis fills with blood, which is then trapped inside vein-like structures. If there is narrowing of the arteries to the penis, erection will not occur. For the penis, clitoris, and vagina to be aroused, they must have an adequate blood supply from the penile and vaginal arteries. If these arteries are compromised, arousal will be incomplete. Some couples find that having sex in non-traditional positions may put pressure on one partner's groin, compromising blood flow to the genitalia, resulting in failure to be aroused, or conversely, that non-traditional positions alleviate groin pressure. Couples with compromised arteries or veins should know that certain positions are more likely to result in one or both partners achieving and maintaining arousal. Older people and men and women with PD have difficulty moving and turning in bed because of rigidity of their muscles, stiffness of their joints, or pain from osteoporotic bones. Some PD patients have found it helpful to take their PD drugs an hour before having sex so that their muscles perform optimally. Silk or satin sheets (or pajamas) may also increase mobility in bed. Some couples use a heated pool where the relative absence of gravity increases their mobility.

Few men bring the issue of erectile dysfunction up with their doctor and few doctors ask about it. This doesn't mean it's not important.

Few men bring the issue of erectile dysfunction up with their doctor and few doctors ask about it. This doesn't mean it's not important. The inability to achieve and maintain an erection is frustrating, embarrassing, and distressing to men and their partners. Achieving and maintaining an erection results from the successful interplay of several different physical and psychological processes. One or more of these may be impaired in PD. Thus, anxiety and/or depression may result in a loss of desire to have or think about sex. The desire to have sex or think about sex is called libido. A loss of libido can result in impotence. Most men with PD, however, retain their desire for sex (as do most women with PD), and this, coupled with impotence or an inability to be aroused, heightens frustration, results in abstinence, and can deepen social isolation.

PD usually begins around age 60, a time when some men and women experience lack of arousal related to any number of reasons, including age, diabetes, an enlarged prostate, Peyronie's disease, depression, or drugs, especially anti-cholinergics, alpha blockers, and beta blockers. Thus, PD itself may not be the cause. Before starting an extensive evaluation, it is important to determine if lack of arousal is physical or psychological. If discussing lack of arousal in the presence of the partner is embarrassing, the patient should initially talk to their doctor alone. But both patient and partner should recognize that an inability to talk openly with one another can add to the problem.

If PD is the reason for inability to achieve arousal, the culprit of PD is ANS insufficiency. Although there are no specific treatments to restore the ANS, careful attention to the drugs a person is taking is helpful. Anti-hypertensives, anti-cholinergics, alpha blockers, and beta blockers all can block arousal, while commonly prescribed PD drugs that act on the dopamine system (levodopa/carbidopa, selegiline, ropinirole) do not. In moderation, alcohol can increase desire and arousal by repressing social inhibitions. However, excess alcohol has the opposite effect. If lack of arousal occurs within a few days of starting a new drug or increasing the dose of an old drug, the drug may be responsible and stopping or lowering the dose may help.

Anxiety, depression, fatigue, and loss of self-esteem can all cause lack of desire and/or arousal in PD patients. Anxiety and depression should be identified, discussed with a partner, and treated. Loss of self-esteem may be related to stooped posture, moving slowly, or tremor. When appearance is a concern it should be discussed with the partner; usually it is more of a concern to the patient than the partner.

In my experience, folk remedies for arousal ("aphrodisiacs") fail to work. Although there are several treatments for lack of arousal, drugs that block an enzyme that causes the arteries to constrict are the most successful and popular. These include Viagra, Cialis, and Levitra. These drugs work by increasing the amount of nitrous oxide, a naturally-occurring chemical. Consult with your doctor to discuss taking one of these medications, proper doses, and potential side effects.

51. I have Parkinson disease—why me?

No one has an answer to "Why me?" It certainly is not anything that you did or didn't do, or anything that you had any control over; thus, you cannot blame yourself. You may wonder why you didn't see it coming, or how and why those early symptoms were never recognized for what they really were. Nothing can turn back the clock or change reality. If you continue to blame yourself, ask your doctor to check to see whether you are depressed. For some people, just having a diagnosis is sufficient. Then they can sit down and discuss the prognosis and start learning as much as they can about PD. Others, especially those who have a relative with PD, may assume the worst and imagine that they will soon be disabled. Some people may be a bit too optimistic, confident that their doctor can make PD disappear with a few prescriptions. After all, we live in a time of great scientific advances, when the contributions of technology to our lives have never been greater. How is it possible, they reason, that PD won't soon be cured? Obviously, a balance between unremitting pessimism and unbridled optimism must be struck.

52. What can I do to cope?

PD does impose major lifestyle changes, and it is easy to feel an overwhelming sense of loss. You can no longer do many things as easily as you did before, or perhaps you may not be able to do them at all. Although PD may define what you can and cannot do, it does not define you. You are not your disease. You can regain a measure of control by making a list of all of the things that you can do. Then make another list of all the things that you can do to care of yourself, such as diet, exercise, managing stress, and taking your drugs on time. Perhaps one of the most difficult hurdles is learning to accept help from others. Because PD will make you unable to do certain things, you will need help. Learn to accept help gracefully, without losing your dignity. Giving help has its own rewards, one of which is an offer of appreciation.

You are not your disease. You can regain a measure of control by making a list of all of the things that you can do.

Another difficulty is responding to the unkind looks or remarks from others, particularly strangers. Although they may never have known anyone with PD, their rudeness or pity is unwelcome. Education—improving public awareness and media coverage or making information about PD available to others—is important. If you have the opportunity and the courage, you could explain to them that you have a neurologic disorder that affects your walking and balance. The Parkinson Disease Society of Great Britain has a small card that can be handed to people that states: "I have Parkinson disease. I may be slow to move or unsteady on my feet. I may have difficulty speaking and writing clearly. I can hear and understand you. Please allow time."

Staying active and interacting with others gives opportunities for expanding your horizons and staying in touch with others. Find, join, and attend PD support groups, which offer camaraderie with other folks who have gone down the same path as you, who know how PD feels, and who can share with you their best methods of coping. They are also an excellent source of knowledge about PD and can keep you posted on the best books and web pages or the newest developments in research and treatment of PD. Friends made in support groups can keep you from feeling alone in your circumstances.

As symptoms progress, it will be necessary to revise your expectations of yourself. Insisting on doing things or driving yourself to places the way that you used to will bring on increased stress and anxiety. Your successes and accomplishments prior to having PD are not realistic goals now. Adjust your priorities accordingly. Set goals for yourself that are attainable and challenging, but that can be accomplished within your physical and emotional limits. Remember past successes, as those memories can be inspiring when you don't feel encouraged. Focus on small victories, and keep track of them. Reward yourself as you meet each goal. Progress will also keep your spirits up and keep you feeling in control of your life. Your accomplishments will bolster your self-esteem.

53. Who do I tell and what should I tell them?

People wonder whom they should tell about their PD, but there are no "right" or "wrong" answers. Sometimes people tell everyone they know, but others tell only the people who are closest to them. PD affects not only the person who has it, but everyone who is close to that person. Trying to hide PD may make the situation worse, adding to the anxiety, especially as the symptoms worsen and are no longer easily concealed. Telling family and friends can be difficult, but not telling them can also cause anxiety. Who and when to tell are decisions that you will need to make, but hearing the news from you is better than having your family and friends guess about what is wrong with you.

PD affects both partners in a relationship. It is important to share the diagnosis with your partner as soon as possible. Facing your partner's reactions may be one of the most difficult challenges of PD. If the relationship is already shaky, the diagnosis of PD may be all that is needed to bring it to an end. But even if the relationship is on a firm foundation, a partner may still have negative reactions, denying the illness or feeling anger about how it will change the relationship. Some partners may become overprotective and smother the person with PD with too much care. Even if you have a great relationship, PD will strain it. Talk to each other—often, and about everything. Good communication is what makes the difference and will make a good relationship an even better one.

Sooner or later your children or grandchildren will need to be told. How you tell them will affect how they deal with both you and PD. Try not to let your anxiety show. Let them know that it is a "natural" event, and reassure them that it isn't fatal or something contagious that they can "catch." Use language that is appropriate for their age and level of understanding. Encourage them to ask questions and share their concerns. The more accepting you are of your condition, the more accepting the children will be, too. In Michael J. Fox's memoir, *Lucky Man* (Hyperion: April 2002), the actor recounts explaining to his five-year-old son about his PD: "Clearly, to Sam, I was still 'Dad,' just 'Dad with the wiggly hand.' Was it possible that I could look at things the same way, that I was still me—just me plus Parkinson?" When you are ready to inform your children or grandchildren of your PD, you may be surprised—as Fox was—at the inspiration that can be drawn from this difficult moment.

People wonder about whether to tell their boss. This depends on several factors and especially on what kind

"Clearly, to Sam, I was still 'Dad,' just 'Dad with the wiggly hand.' Was it possible that I could look at things the same way, that I was still me—just me plus Parkinson?"

of job you have and your relationship with your boss. Will PD affect your job performance? An airline pilot or a surgeon will have to tell his or her employer sooner than someone who works in sales. How your boss responds may not be predictable either. Although PD is a disability and federal law prohibits firing a person because of a disability, you could be reassigned to a different job or be pressured into taking early retirement. Then again, an employer might be willing to make accommodations to keep you or even allow you to work from home. For many people, their job helps them to feel defined—what they do is who they are. Finding yourself without your occupational definition of self—regardless of how gently you are let go or with what allowances—can be a terrible blow. Finding another way to use your skills and knowledge will lead to new ways of being productive and can restore your sense of identity. Other people may be close enough to retirement when they are diagnosed with PD that they are grateful for the excuse to retire and do things that they have waited for years to do.

54. Will I still be able to drive?

Driving is the one common ritual that measures maturity and independence. As a teen, getting a driver's license is a major milestone of independence. Giving up driving is, for some people, equivalent to losing their freedom and independence. Can a person with PD continue to drive?

Early in PD, driving should pose no problem as long as symptoms are mild and don't interfere with your ability to react to traffic situations. As symptoms progress, however, decreased motor skills and concentration may compromise your ability to drive. When muscle rigidity and lack of coordination make it difficult to react quickly, the reality of the situation must be faced, and the decision to drive must be reconsidered. The spouse or care-partner or one of the children, not the patient, usually raises the question about driving. It is a rare patient who voluntarily gives up driving. I ask the spouse if she or he feels comfortable driving with the patient or if she or he feels comfortable with the patient driving the grandchildren. I also ask about recent accidents. A recent history of several accidents, even relatively minor ones, signals a problem driving. If there is any question about driving skills and abilities, a professional driving instructor can evaluate the situation.

A loss of driving does not necessarily mean a loss of independence or isolation: not driving doesn't mean not going places. Take stock of all of the available options: a partner who is happy to drive, a friend who is willing to accompany you to appointments, and public transportation. If you no longer have the expense of maintaining a car and insurance, the price of a taxi ride is a bargain. It may take a bit more planning to arrange, but don't give up on going places just because you can't drive.

55. How will my social life change?

Staying connected with other people is vital. It is easy to feel embarrassed about the symptoms of PD and withdraw, but this only leads to isolation and depression. When you give in to PD, you become its victim, suffering embarrassment and loneliness. When you accept that PD is a reality in your life, you can find ways of coping, thus regaining a sense of control and getting on with living your life. Remaining active with social events, going to church, going to the theater or concerts, and entertaining at home may take a bit

Staying connected with other people is vital.

more effort, but is worth it. It is important to interact with others and to share your thoughts, hopes, and dreams. Join a gym and exercise regularly—it will help you stay in shape as well as get you out with other people. Take up yoga; it will calm your mind as you stretch and keep your muscles limber. Members of a support group offer camaraderie and will share their own methods of coping.

56. As a care-partner, how can I cope with my partner's Parkinson disease?

As a partner of someone with PD, you never expected to be in this situation, and you may feel unprepared for your new responsibilities. Frustration, anger, resentment, fear, sadness, and hopelessness may all rush over you, and then you may feel guilty for having these emotions! Life seems to be spinning out of control. Like your PD partner, you need to accept this situation because PD is something over which you have no control. When you accept this, you can focus on parts of your life over which you do have control, where you can establish some kind of order and impose some kind of schedule to regain a saner perspective. The balance of your relationship is shifting; you will be challenged emotionally, spiritually, and physically. A partner who mowed the lawn and kept the garden may no longer be able to perform these tasks. A partner who shopped and cooked and cleaned the house may have to share those tasks with his or her mate. At times, the responsibility for the home combined with care-giving for the ill partner can become so burdensome that you feel pushed beyond your abilities to cope.

As a care-partner you must take care of yourself physically by eating a balanced diet and getting enough sleep and regular exercise. Exercise is a great way to relieve stress while strengthening you for the physical challenges of being a care-partner. Take care of yourself emotionally by learning to channel your emotions and feelings into constructive outlets. Find a support group for care-partners. Talk about your feelings with friends and family. Learn as much about PD as possible so that the next challenge won't come as such a surprise. Take time to do the things that you enjoy: go for a walk or spend time with nature or meet a friend for lunch. Don't neglect your spiritual side either; connect with your higher power and meditate or pray every day. Let your spirituality give you strength.

When your workload feels impossible, it probably is. Rally your resources, gather family and friends to give you a hand, or check on resources that are available in your community. Hire some help so that your time is spent where it is needed most. Maybe you need to adjust your expectations a bit—you may be setting too high a standard for yourself. Perfection is not necessary and a burned-out caregiver is not able to care for anyone.

To be a good care-partner sometimes means allowing the person with PD to be independent. It may be easier and faster for you to do something, but remember that your partner may still be able to do many things—it just takes longer. Encourage him or her to be independent and active and to do as much as possible independently. There may be times when the best you can do is merely to be there, to sit beside your partner, hold hands, or lend your moral support.

To be a good care-partner sometimes means allowing the person with PD to be independent.

PART FIVE

The Next Six to Thirty Years After Diagnosis

What is levodopa/carbidopa?

What are Comtan, Stalevo, and Tasmar?

What are symptoms of depression in Parkinson disease and how is it treated?

More . . .

57. What is levodopa/carbidopa?

Levodopa/carbidopa, or Sinemet (the brand name for levodopa/carbidopa), treats most of the symptoms of PD. It's the most powerful anti-Parkinson drug on the market. However, after 2 to 5 years it usually causes "wearing-off," a loss of effectiveness of a dose before the next dose is due, like the battery of your computer giving out before you have a chance to change it. Wearing off results in the re-emergence of Parkinson symptoms with the symptoms persisting despite your taking the next dose of levodopa/carbidopa. As the effectiveness of each dose of levodopa/carbidopa gets shorter and you take the drug more frequently, you develop dyskinesias: abnormal involuntary, uncontrollable "dance-like" movements. The emergence of wearing off and dyskinesia has prompted some experts to question whether levodopa/carbidopa might damage the remaining cells in the substantia nigra. The levodopa in levodopa/carbidopa is changed by into dopamine the cells in the substantia nigra. As PD progresses, these neurons becomes less effective in changing levodopa to dopamine, requiring ever more frequent and higher amounts of levodopa/carbidopa. Because the appearance of wearing off and dyskinesia starts within 2 to 5 years of starting levodopa/carbidopa, it is usually withheld as long as possible, and the underlying deficiency of dopamine is treated with dopamine agonists and/or MAO-B inhibitors.

The appearance of wearing off and dyskinesia does not mean levodopa/carbidopa is no longer effective; it is effective as long as there are neurons in the substantia nigra. The early use of levodopa/carbidopa at high doses is more likely to result in wearing-off and dyskinesia. The trick is to use as low a dose of levodopa/carbidopa as possible (less than 600 mg per day) and substitute dopamine agonists and MAO-B inhibitors whenever possible.

Levodopa/carbidopa comes in two forms: a regular release and a controlled release (CR) or extended release (ER) preparation. Regular release levodopa/carbidopa comes in three preparations: 10/100, a 1:10 preparation of carbidopa to levodopa, a 25/250, also a 1:10 preparation of carbidopa to levodopa, and 25/100, a 1:4 preparation of carbidopa to levodopa. The first number stands for the dose of carbidopa, the second number stands for the dose of levodopa. The lower ratio of carbidopa to levodopa, 1 to 4, means there's more carbidopa. Controlled release (CR) or extended release (ER), levodopa/carbidopa comes in two preparations: 25/100, a 1 to 4 preparation of carbidopa to levodopa, and a 50/200, also a 1:4 preparation of carbidopa to levodopa.

58. Are generic drugs as good as brand name drugs?

There are currently several different generic forms of regular and controlled-release levodopa/carbidopa. These generic preparations are cheaper and usually require no copayment. For a generic drug to be approved, it must release the same amount of levodopa as the brand name, but there can be up to a 20% variability. For most people with PD (approximately 70%) the generic drugs are equivalent to the brand name ones, but in up to 30% of patients they are not. It is good to keep in mind that if your doctor writes a prescription for a generic drug, the pharmacist is free to substitute one generic for another, which may create more variability. Generic drugs can be compared to soft drinks in that there are brand name colas (Coke or Pepsi) as well as generic colas. Many people are willing to pay extra for Coke or Pepsi, while others feel the generic cola is fine. Obviously there is a

Generic drugs can be compared to soft drinks in that there are brand name colas (Coke or Pepsi) as well as generic colas.

bigger price difference between brand name drugs and generics than between Coke or Pepsi and generic colas, and most drug benefit plans aren't willing to pay the difference.

59. Does levodopa make Parkinson disease worse?

Levodopa/carbidopa has been the gold standard for PD treatment since it was introduced in 1967, but in the intervening years, due to recognition of its complications (wearing off and dyskinesia), a debate ensued as to whether levodopa/carbidopa should be delayed so as to delay its complications. Before the introduction of dopamine agonists and MAO-B inhibitors, there was no alternative to levodopa/carbidopa. Although less powerful than levodopa/carbidopa, the agonists and MAO-B inhibitors are less likely to result in wearing off and dyskinesia even after levodopa/carbidopa has already been started.

At one time, it was theorized that levodopa might be a factor in the death of dopamine cells, the idea being that the large amount of dopamine formed from levodopa might generate enough free radicals to damage the dopamine neurons. The Elldopa study, initiated by Dr. Stan Fahn and the Parkinson Study Group, tested the idea. Elldopa was a multi-center, double-blind, dose-ranging, randomized study in which 361 patients with early PD, who did NOT need levodopa/carbidopa, were randomly assigned to one of four treatments, using levodopa/carbidopa or a placebo.

The dose of levodopa/carbidopa was gradually increased over time and then maintained until treatment was stopped. After two weeks without treatment, patients were re-examined using the Unified Parkinson Disease

Rating Scale (UPDRS). All patients who'd been on levodopa/carbidopa had lower UPDRS scores than patients who'd been on placebo. The results suggest that levodopa is effective in a dose-dependent manner in treating the symptoms of PD and may slow its progression, though one must be cautious in this latter suggestion. Although there are limitations in the Elldopa Study, the central result stands: levodopa does NOT make PD worse. Although levodopa does not make PD worse, its early use is more likely to result in wearing off and dyskinesias and in most patients should be started only after first using a dopamine agonist and/or an MAO-B inhibitor.

60. Why is carbidopa combined with levodopa?

When levodopa was introduced, its main side effects were nausea and vomiting. In spite of its benefits, many patients couldn't or wouldn't take it. The problem was in the conversion of levodopa to dopamine. The levodopa was converted into dopamine in the stomach, liver, kidneys, and blood by an enzyme called dopa-decarboxylase (DDC). Dopamine in the blood reacts with the body's vomiting center to cause nausea and vomiting. The vomiting center is partly in the brain (inside the blood-brain barrier) and partly outside the brain. To stop levodopa from being converted to dopamine outside the brain in the periphery, carbidopa is used to block the enzyme DDC. Carbidopa does not cross the blood-brain barrier and thus does not block the conversion of levodopa to dopamine inside the brain. Adding carbidopa prevents the nausea that's associated with levodopa and allows an approximately 80% decrease in the dose of levodopa. The name Sinemet was chosen for the preparation of levodopa/carbidopa because Sinemet means "no vomiting"—in Latin "sine" means without, and "emit" means vomiting.

61. Why is there a regular and a controlled release (CR) levodopa/carbidopa?

Levodopa/carbidopa comes as regular release and a controlled (CR) or extended release (ER) preparation. People with advanced PD who had prominent wearing off were expected to benefit from a CR preparation of levodopa/carbidopa. Levodopa is absorbed from the small bowel after passing through the stomach, but the coating surrounding CR slows both the release of levodopa from the stomach and its absorption from the small bowel. Although CR is helpful, it hasn't lived up to its expectations. It takes one hour for regular release levodopa/carbidopa to achieve a peak effect and this peak is usually high enough to turn patients "on." The effect of regular release levodopa lasts two hours. In early PD, the brain is able to store dopamine and, although the blood levels of levodopa drop, the stored dopamine is enough to "ride out" the shortfall. Although blood levels from CR last twice as long as those from regular release levodopa/carbidopa, the levels usually never achieve a high enough peak to turn patients on.

A myth about CR is that if you break it in half, or if you crush it, it's not effective, but this is false.

A myth about CR is that if you break it in half, or if you crush it, it's not effective, but this is false. If you break CR in half the exposed surfaces are no longer surrounded by the coating and you lose about 10% of CR's effect. If you crush the CR tablet, it acts like a regular release tablet. CR is often used as an adjunct to regular release levodopa/carbidopa. Sometimes the regular and CR tablets are given together so that the peak effect of the regular release tablet can turn the patient on, while CR maintains the on period. Sometimes CR is given at night to prevent patients from wearing off during the night. Combining regular release levodopa/carbidopa with Tasmar or Comtan in Stalevo is more effective than combining regular release and CR in achieving a peak and a long duration effect. It's thought that wearing off and dyskinesias are less likely to occur if blood levels of levodopa are constant. Before you had PD, the neurons in your putamen, the target of the neurons in your substantia nigra, "saw" dopamine continuously. After you develop PD they see dopamine intermittently. The closer you can approximate the situation before you had PD, the less likely you'll have wearing off. Such continuous stimulation can be approximated by a combination of dopamine agonists, MAO-B inhibitors, levodopa/carbidopa 4 times a day, and Comtan or Tasmar.

To increase the effectiveness of levodopa/carbidopa, it's important to take it approximately half an hour before eating, as the volume of the food in your stomach, and in some people the protein content of their food, may slow or block the absorption of levodopa from the small bowel. You want to get levodopa as quickly as possible from your stomach, where it may be broken down, into your small bowel where it's absorbed. Food slows down the passage of levodopa through your stomach.

62. What are Comtan, Stalevo, and Tasmar?

Comtan, alone or in Stalevo, blocks an enzyme called COMT. COMT is present both inside and outside cells, so it is able to circulate in the blood. Comtan blocks COMT, but as it does not enter the brain, it can't block COMT there. Another COMT inhibitor, Tasmar, blocks COMT both inside and outside the brain. Comtan and Tasmar are effective ways to prolong the actions of levodopa/carbidopa by making more levodopa available to the brain. They are more effective in prolonging the actions of levodopa/carbidopa than controlled release levodopa/carbidopa.

Comtan and Tasmar work differently from Zelapar or Azilect; however, these medications complement each other. Zelapar and Azilect preserve the dopamine formed from levodopa inside the brain. Comtan and Tasmar make more of the "raw material" levodopa available, while Zelapar and Azilect utilize the product of the raw material dopamine more efficiently.

Some neurologists will start patients on Comtan as soon as they start levodopa/carbidopa. Others start Comtan when patients begin to develop wearing off. The addition of Comtan results in a more continuous delivery of levodopa to the brain, which more closely resembles the situation in the brain before the patient developed PD.

Comtan (generic name entacapone) can be added to levodopa/carbidopa (in a dose of 200 mg) or can be combined with levodopa/carbidopa in a single tablet, called Stalevo. Stalevo is usually given three times a day, 30 minutes to an hour before meals. Comtan prolongs the half-life of levodopa, so the benefits of Comtan or Stalevo are similar to the benefits of levodopa, with the exception that by prolonging the duration of levodopa they decrease the wearing off.

The side effects of Comtan are similar to the adverse effects of levodopa, including dyskinesia. Two effects of Comtan (and Tasmar) separate from levodopa are diarrhea (5% of patients) and dark yellowish discoloration of the urine. If diarrhea occurs, Comtan or Tasmar should be stopped, but levodopa can be continued.

Comtan is given with each dose of levodopa/carbidopa. Tasmar is given three times a day, regardless of the number of doses of levodopa/carbidopa. As a rule, Tasmar is more effective in prolonging the actions of levodopa than Comtan. However, because a small number of patients may develop liver failure on Tasmar, all patients on Tasmar must be closely monitored with tests of liver function. This requirement has limited the use of Tasmar.

63. What are Parcopa and Madopar?

Parcopa is a preparation of levodopa/carbidopa that dissolves in your mouth, is transported to your stomach, and is then absorbed in your small bowel. Parcopa can be carried in your pocket and taken without water, if you need an extra dose of drug. I use it when I test patients' responses to levodopa. In patients who are uncertain if they are responding to levodopa, I ask them to stop levodopa for at least 24 hours, evaluate them off levodopa, then give them a test of Parcopa, and evaluate them an hour later. Parcopa works faster than levodopa/carbidopa, especially if you chew it before swallowing it. Chewing Parcopa breaks up the tablet, creating a larger surface area, and allowing the tablet to pass more quickly from the stomach into the small bowel where it's absorbed.

Madopar or Madopa or Prolopa (the name of Madopar in Canada) is a combination of levodopa and benserazide (a DDC inhibitor). Like levodopa/carbidopa, Madopar is available in a 25/100 preparation: 25 mg of benserazide and 100 mg of levodopa. About 20% of patients do better on levodopa/carbidopa, 20% do better on Madopar, and 60% do just as well on either drug. Madopar is not available in the United States, but can be obtained from Canada through a doctor's prescription. If you're unable to tolerate levodopa/carbidopa, ask your doctor if you might benefit

The Next Six to Thirty Years After Diagnosis

from Madopar. Since it's not a U.S. drug, your drug benefit plan will not pay for it.

64. What is liquid levodopa/carbidopa?

Some patients with advanced PD who're having wearing off and dyskinesia on levodopa/carbidopa may benefit from "liquid" levodopa/carbidopa. In these patients, a tablet of levodopa/carbidopa 25/100 is too much: they "turn on" but develop dyskinesia. However, a half tablet of levodopa/carbidopa, 12.5/50 is too little. I tell such patients to dissolve a single 25/100 tablet in 100 ml of water. The tablet doesn't dissolve completely; it forms a suspension. I tell patients to mix the suspension with Tang, which has a high vitamin C content and makes the suspension more uniform. The suspension allows patients to control the amount of medication they consume, only drinking as much as is needed. Once you've found the dose of levodopa that "turns you on" with a minimal amount of dyskinesias, you can prepare a daily suspension of levodopa/ carbidopa (with Tang) and take the dose of levodopa that best fits your needs. A preparation of liquid levodopa/carbidopa called Dou-dopa is available. This preparation is administered through a tube directly into the small bowel (the duodenum) and provides a nearly constant level of levodopa in the blood and in the brain. The insertion of the tube is a surgical procedure. Dou-dopa is for patients with intolerable wearing off who aren't candidates for deep brain stimulation.

65. What is apomorphine?

Apomorphine is a dopamine agonist that is rapidly broken down, or metabolized, in the liver. It's almost impossible to achieve high blood levels of apomorphine by taking the drug orally due to its rapid metabolism in the liver. However, apomorphine can be injected under your skin (subcutaneously), which bypasses your liver and results in high and sustained levels of apomorphine in your blood. Apokyn is the name of an injectible preparation of apomorphine used to reverse your "off" periods. Apokyn may, initially be tricky to use, so a doctor or a nurse will teach you how to use it. If you inject too little you don't "turn on," but if you inject too much you may become nauseated, vomit, or may experience orthostatic hypotension. Some patients, prior to injecting themselves with Apokyn, take an anti-nauseant such as Tigan (an anti-histamine) or domperidone (available in Canada and Europe). Although many patients achieve remarkable benefits from Apokyn, the problems of learning to inject yourself and the need for daily injections has limited Apokyn's use.

66. What is wearing-off?

"Wearing off" is defined as the gradual loss of effectiveness of a given dose of levodopa/carbidopa before the next dose is due. Similarly, "on-off" is defined as the abrupt or sudden loss of effectiveness of a given dose of levodopa/carbidopa before the next dose is due. The mechanisms underlying "wearing off" and "on-off" are similar—and the terms are often used synonymously.

Wearing off and on-off result in part from:

• *The short duration of levodopa's action.* Levodopa has a peak effect in an hour. The **half-life** of levodopa is 2 hours, which means that it takes two hours for the peak dose of levodopa to fall by 50%. It takes 5 half-lives for a drug to be cleared from the blood. So if you take a dose of levodopa/carbidopa, there will be

The mechanisms underlying "wearing off" and "on-off" are similar— and the terms are often used synonymously.

Half-life

A measure of the duration of the drug's action.

detectable levels of levodopa in your blood 10 hours later, but these levels are not enough to turn you "on," or prevent you from going "off." The short duration of levodopa's action means that levodopa has a pulsatile (rather than continuous) effect—such pulsatile effects predispose you to develop wearing off and dyskinesia. If you can increase the half life of a dose of levodopa by combining it with a drug such as Comtan (present in Stalevo) or Tasmar, or with an MAO-B inhibitor such as rasagiline or selegiline, you decrease the chances of levodopa wearing off.

- *A delay in the passage of levodopa from the stomach into the small bowel.* Levodopa is broken down by the enzyme DDC in the wall of the stomach and part of the dose may not reach the small bowel. Food slows the passage of levodopa, so if you take levodopa with food, more levodopa is "broken-down" and less reaches the brain. In patients who are protein sensitive, protein-rich foods hinder the absorption of levodopa from the small bowel. Such patients quickly learn to avoid protein-rich foods during the day and take most of their protein in a single meal at night. As PD advances, the stomach loses some of its elasticity and doesn't empty as well or as promptly as before; this may also contribute to wearing off. In my experience, 20% of wearing off is related to taking levodopa/carbidopa during meals or with protein-rich food.

- *Changes in the sensitivity of the dopamine receptors on the neurons in the putamen* (the target of the neurons in the substantia nigra). The principal cause of wearing off is a change in the sensitivity of the dopamine receptors. The receptors are proteins, living molecules that adapt to the changing conditions of PD. Before you had PD, these receptors "saw" dopamine all the time, as enough dopamine was being made by the neurons in your substantia nigra. After you developed PD and became dependent on a sporadically delivered outside source of dopamine (levodopa), some of the receptors over-reacted to dopamine, resulting in dyskinesia, and some of the receptors didn't react, resulting in wearing off.

Minimizing the wearing off effect involves:

- *Starting treatment with a dopamine agonist or an MAO-B inhibitor.* However, patients 75 years of age and older do not tolerate dopamine agonists as well as they tolerate levodopa/carbidopa and are more likely to develop drowsiness and mental changes.
- *Adding Comtan (in Stalevo) or Tasmar to levodopa/ carbidopa.* These drugs increase the half life of levodopa by approximately 50%.
- *Taking levodopa/carbidopa at least half an hour before meals* (and avoiding protein-rich meals if you're protein sensitive). To increase the effectiveness of levodopa/carbidopa, it's important to take it approximately half an hour before eating, as the volume of the food in your stomach may slow or block the absorption of levodopa from the small bowel. You want to get levodopa as quickly as possible from your stomach, where it may be broken down, into your small bowel where it's absorbed.

67. How do I know if I am under- or over-medicated?

Patients frequently wonder whether certain symptoms are related to PD or to the medications they take to treat PD. Generally, symptoms such as slowness of movement, tremor, rigidity or stiffness, and difficulty walking are all symptoms that were present before treatment for PD began and so are related to PD. Symptoms such as dyskinesia are, as a rule, related to the effects of PD drugs. There are other symptoms that can be related to PD and/or can be aggravated by PD drugs, thus making it difficult to determine the cause. These symptoms include dystonia, confusion, disorientation, and shortness of breath.

Dystonia, a painful cramping of the legs or arms, occurs in people with PD before they're treated, yet the same symptom can be due to aggravation by PD drugs. Confusion, disorientation, delusions, hallucinations and abnormal behavior all occur in PD patients who are evolving a dementia. Yet these symptoms can also be caused by PD drugs. Shortness of breath occurs in some PD patients because the muscles of the chest wall are rigid and don't move well, indicating a need for additional doses of levodopa. The same symptom, however, can occur because of dyskinesia of the chest wall muscles, indicating too much levodopa. The following rules are helpful in determining if a symptom is related to PD or to the drugs for PD:

- If the symptom begins shortly after a new drug is added or an old drug is increased, the symptom may be related to the drug.
- If the symptom was there before a new drug is added or an old drug is increased, the symptom is probably disease-related.
- If there is doubt as to whether the symptom is related to PD or the drug, then with your doctor's approval decrease the dose of the drug. If the symptom decreases or disappears it was likely drug-related. How much to decrease the drug, and how rapidly, is an issue that must be discussed with your doctor.

Keep track of how you are doing. Each week, and especially after a change is made in a drug, or after a new drug is added, fill out the Activities of Daily Living part of the UPDRS. The total score isn't as important as a change in a particular activity. In addition, you should keep track of your handwriting on a weekly basis. At the Muhammad Ali Parkinson Center we recommend you write a sentence, in script, on a single line. We recommend the sentence "This is a sample of my best handwriting." If your handwriting becomes larger, or there is more space between the words and letters, it may indicate improvement. If your handwriting becomes smaller and there is less space between the words and letters, your symptoms may be getting worse. If you take medication for diabetes, you learn to check your glucose levels. Similarly, if you are on drugs for PD, you should complete the ADL chart and keep track of your handwriting on a regular basis.

Keep track of how you are doing. Each week, and especially after a change is made in a drug, or after a new drug is added, fill out the Activities of Daily Living part of the UPDRS.

68. What are dyskinesias?

Dyskinesias, or chorea from the Greek word meaning dance, as in choreography, are irregular, non-rhythmical, dance-like, uncontrolled involuntary movements. Dyskinesia differs from the regular, rhythm-like involuntary movement that is tremor. Dyskinesia may involve the head, neck, trunk, arms and legs and are usually more marked on the side most severely affected by PD, which is usually the side on which PD began. Dyskinesia may or may not be associated with dystonia—a prolonged and often painful spasm of a limb. When dyskinesia and dystonia appear together it may be difficult to distinguish them.

Dyskinesias vary in amplitude, duration, and in body parts affected. Dyskinesias of the head can result in "bobbing," turning, or twisting movements of the head and neck. Dyskinesias of the face can result in grimacing, eye blinking, nose twitching, lip smacking, or in the tongue darting in-and-out of the mouth. Dyskinesias of the trunk can result in the body swaying or rocking to-and-fro. In some patients, dyskinesia affects the intercostal muscles and diaphragm, which can result in irregular respirations, with the patient complaining of shortness of breath. Dyskinesias of the pelvis can result in thrusting, lewd-like movements of the hips, pelvis, and lower spine. Finally, dyskinesias of the arms and legs can result in an inability to use them, or an inability to walk.

Dyskinesias are not part of PD itself, but rather they result from the effects of levodopa on a brain that has become sensitized to levodopa because of PD. Thus, patients with diseases other than PD, such as dopa responsive dystonia, restless legs syndrome, or multiple system atrophy and are treated with levodopa do not develop dyskinesias. Dyskinesias are more common in younger PD patients because older patients are not usually treated with the same high dose of levodopa as younger patients. In addition, the brains of younger patients are more sensitive to levodopa.

Dyskinesias usually appear after two or more years of treatment with levodopa. The higher the dose of levodopa and the longer the duration of treatment, the more likely dyskinesias will develop. Dyskinesias usually appear $1/2$ to 1 $1/2$ hours after a dose of levodopa as levels of levodopa peak, called "peak dose dyskinesia." Here, a high blood and brain level of levodopa triggers the dyskinesia. In about 25% of PD patients, dyskinesia appears within a few minutes of taking levodopa, or two or more hours after taking levodopa, as the levels of levodopa fall. These are called "di-phasic dyskinesias."

The mechanism of di-phasic dyskinesia probably results from an abrupt fall in levodopa levels. Patients with both "peak dose" and "di-phasic dyskinesias" are difficult to treat: because of the different mechanisms responsible for the dyskinesias.

Initially, most patients started on levodopa as their first PD drug have a 2- to 5-year "grace period" or "levodopa honeymoon." During this period, a dose to levodopa/carbidopa of 100 mg of levodopa and 25 mg of carbidopa, 3 to 4 times a day, results in good control of your PD symptoms (an exception may be tremor). You may even miss a dose or two, or a day of levodopa/carbidopa without re-emergence of your PD symptoms. Presumably, you have enough neurons in your substantia nigra to change levodopa to dopamine, to deliver dopamine to receptors in your putamen, and to store some dopamine as a reserve. Gradually, however, as PD progresses, you lose neurons in your substantia nigra and the remaining neurons have to work harder, you increase the frequency and the amount of your levodopa. This, in turn, results in dyskinesia.

69. What is the most levodopa/carbidopa I can take?

The levodopa in carbidopa/levodopa is a "pro-drug," meaning it must be changed in the brain into dopamine. Unlike blood sugar, the blood dopa level is not a guide as to how much dopamine the brain needs (this is why blood dopa levels are not done routinely). In the early 1970s, after carbidopa/levodopa was introduced (but before the agonists), doctors gave enough levodopa, usually 400–1,200 mg per day, to bring out dyskinesia. The presence of mild dyskinesia, it was reasoned, indicated the brain had enough dopamine. However, in time, mild dyskinesia, without the addition

Unlike blood sugar, the blood dopa level is not a guide as to how much dopamine the brain needs.

of more levodopa, became marked dyskinesia. Subsequently, doctors gave lower doses of levodopa. But because levodopa is short acting, patients eventually developed "wearing off" and many developed dyskinesia. Most patients preferred dyskinesia to wearing off. In part, they preferred being mobile (even hyper-mobile) to being immobile; in part because "wearing off" was often associated with discomfort and/or pain, whereas dyskinesia was not; and in part because some patients became euphoric or "high" when "on" and anxious, depressed, or panicky when "off." In most patients, the dose of carbidopa/levodopa is kept below 1,000 mg. However, some patients exceed this dose.

70. What is the connection between neuroleptic malignant syndrome and levodopa holidays?

Neuroleptic malignant syndrome (NMS) is an unusual reaction to neuroleptic drugs (drugs used as major tranquilizers) and to the abrupt withdrawal of levodopa after several years of treatment. Neuroleptic drugs block dopamine receptors in the brain and, for reasons that remain unclear, in a small group of patients, NMS results. The treatment of NMS in these patients is to stop the offending neuroleptic and add a dopamine agonist. In some patients, when levodopa is abruptly withdrawn after several years of treatment, the dopamine receptors, sensing their lack of stimulation, act as though they are blocked and NMS develops.

In the past, when levodopa was the only drug available for PD, levodopa holidays (abrupt withdrawal of levodopa) were used when patients developed side effects like delusions, hallucinations, and dyskinesias. For some of these patients, the "holiday" resulted in NMS, characterized by high fever, unresponsiveness, rigidity, and autonomic nervous system dysfunction. These symptoms usually developed a few days after stopping levodopa.

The mortality rate associated with unrecognized and untreated NMS is at least 10%. The key is timely and proper diagnosis. NMS must be considered if symptoms develop after abruptly stopping levodopa. Treatment consists of reintroduction of levodopa and/or addition of a dopamine agonist, and supportive care.

71. What is the connection between levodopa and melanoma?

Some researchers feel there is a possible relationship between Parkinson disease, a disorder of decreased neuromelanin in the brain, and melanoma, a pigmented (or non-pigmented) malignant tumor of the skin (and body). Melanoma contains an enzyme, tyrosine oxidase, that uses levodopa as an energy source, hence the question of a relationship between melanoma and PD. Based on this question, a note of caution was sounded regarding the use of levodopa in PD. A warning in the *Physician's Desk Reference* (a guide that doctors use in determining which drugs might be used for treating a condition) first appeared in 1976 (and continues) for Sinemet, which read:

Because levodopa may activate a malignant melanoma, it should not be used in patients with suspicious, undiagnosed skin lesions or a history of inflammation.

However, no definitive answer has been found to this question and, at present, the evidence for a link between levodopa and recurrence of melanoma is anecdotal and not well documented. In addition, many people with both PD and a history of melanoma have been successfully treated with levodopa without a recurrence of their melanoma. Dopamine agonists such as Mirapex, Requip, and Neupro may be considered as alternatives to levodopa in PD patients with melanoma.

72. What are the symptoms of depression in Parkinson disease and how is it treated?

In PD, in addition to the loss of dopamine cells in the substantia nigra, there are losses of dopamine, noradrenalin, and serotonin neurons in other regions of the brain, including the mesocortical and mesolimbic regions. The dopamine, noradrenalin, and serotonin neurons of the mesocortical and mesolimbic regions originate in the brainstem, in the vicinity of the substantia nigra, and project to centers on the inner surface of the brain. Changes in and/or loss of neurons in these regions may result in the depression and anxiety that often accompany PD.

Depression is characterized by the presence of a majority of the following symptoms:

- Depressed mood most of the day, nearly every day, as indicated by either subjective report (e.g., feels sad or empty) or observation made by others (e.g., appears tearful). This may include feelings of isolation, hopelessness, loneliness, and chronic pain (with or without known cause).
- Significant weight gain or weight loss when not dieting, or increase/decrease in daily appetite.
- Insomnia or excessive sleepiness nearly every day.
- Psychomotor agitation or retardation nearly every day. This may include anxiety, anger, hostility, acting-out, irritability, delusions, hallucinations, paranoia, or psychotic behavior.

- Fatigue or loss of energy nearly every day.
- Feelings of worthlessness or excessive or inappropriate guilt or shame nearly every day.
- Diminished ability to think or concentrate, or indecisiveness, nearly every day.
- Recurrent thoughts of death (not just fear of dying), recurrent suicidal ideation without a specific plan, or a suicide attempt or specific plan for committing suicide.

The severity of depression can by gauged by questionnaires such as the Depression Scale (**see Table 7**). The diagnosis of depression in people with PD can be complicated by an overlap between symptoms of depression and those of PD. For instance, people with PD who move slowly, have an expressionless face, and speak softly may appear depressed when they are not, while depressed people with those same symptoms may appear to have PD when they don't. A structured interview with the patient and caregiver, with the use of a depression questionnaire, can help in diagnosing depression.

Depression may be a reaction to a specific situation such as the loss of a loved one, the loss of a job, loss of self-esteem, and/or being diagnosed with PD. Although depression may be due to an external event, it can affect people with PD as much as tremor, rigidity, and bradykinesia. In fact, depression is common in PD; the lifetime incidence of depression in the general population is estimated to be 16%, while in PD patients it is closer to 48%. Several studies revealed that depression often precedes the diagnosis of PD and that there's a higher rate of depression among people with PD than among people with other diseases and similar degrees of disability.

A structured interview with the patient and caregiver, with the use of a depression questionnaire, can help in diagnosing depression.

Table 7   Depression Scale

For the past week, rate the following symptoms on a scale of:
0 = symptom absent; 1 = symptom mild; 2 = symptom moderate;
3 = symptom marked or severe; 4 = symptom incapacitating

1	Do you feel depressed, discouraged? Do you cry a lot?
2	Do you feel sad, down? Do you think about dying?
3	Do you feel isolated, lonely, hopeless?
4	Do you feel guilty, ashamed, sorry?
5	Are you always in pain or hurting?
6	Have you lost your appetite? Or had a significant weight loss?
7	Do you feel insecure, helpless?

8	Do you LACK the energy to do things?
9	Do you LACK the desire for sex?
10	Do you LACK pleasure in doing things?
11	Do you LACK initiative? Do you fail to take the lead?

12	Do your feel afraid, fearful?
13	Are you UNABLE to concentrate, or pay attention, or remember?
14	Do your moods change RAPIDLY: are you sad than happy?
15	Do you feel anxious? Or worried?
16	Are you Agitated? Irritable? Stubborn?
17	Do you panic easily?

18	Are you UNABLE to fall asleep or stay asleep at night?
19	Do you sleep a lot during the day?
20	Do you feel detached, unreal, not in this world?
21	Do people say bad things about you or try to hurt you?
22	Do you think your spouse or partner is having an affair?

23	Do you SEE or HEAR things that aren't there?
24	Do you have thoughts you can't control? Are you obsessed?
25	Do you, more than before, act on impulse? As an example do you gamble, eat, or shop compulsively?

0–6:	No Depression
7–10:	Mild Depression
11–25:	Moderate—Marked Depression

Anxiety and depression are often thought of as separate disorders. Anxiety is associated with symptoms of "over-activity" of the sympathetic part of the ANS—the part that prepares us for "fight or flight." Depression, however, is associated with symptoms of over-activity of the parasympathetic part of the ANS—the "calming" part, which may become so calm that you are depressed. Although the symptoms of depression and anxiety can be distinguished, they can occur simultaneously. Many people with PD who are depressed are also anxious, and likewise many who are anxious are also depressed. This suggests that both the sympathetic and parasympathetic nervous systems are malfunctioning.

The following are situations characterized by depression mixed with other symptoms or disorders:

Depression and agitation. Depression is usually characterized by silence, withdrawal, and decreased activity. Occasionally, people with PD become agitated and their behavior may indicate an agitated depression. Agitation may also be a symptom of an evolving dementia or the result of changes in the brain caused by high fevers, liver or kidney failure, or medication. These should all be considered before diagnosing an agitated depression.

Depression and sleep disorders. An inability to fall asleep at night, frequent waking during the nights, and excessive drowsiness during the day, are symptoms that often occur in people with PD and depression. It is thought that approximately 50% of people with PD develop a sleep disorder and that an even higher number of PD patients with depression have a co-existing sleep disorder.

Depression and bipolar disorder. Bipolar disorder is a cyclic condition during which people exhibit elevated (manic) and depressive episodes. Most people with bipolar disorder will experience a number of episodes, each lasting three to six months. Ultra-rapid cycling, defined as dramatic mood shifts occurring within a 24- to 48-hour period, occurs in a small number of patients. Such rapid cycling can be induced or made worse by antidepressants unless there is also treatment for the cycling. The relationship of bipolar disorder and PD is unclear (there may or may not be a higher prevalence of PD among people with bipolar disorder) because the rapid cycling of moods resembles the rapid cycling of moods that occur in PD when patients experience wearing off: they are elated when they are "on" and depressed when they are "off."

Depression and dementia. Depressed patients may experience "negative" symptoms, so called because they are characterized by an absence of something. Negative symptoms imply a defect or malfunctioning of the mesocortical and mesolimbic pathways, which modulate behavior and emotion. Negative symptoms include: apathy (lack of motivation or initiative), **anergia** (lack of physical and mental energy), **anhedonia** (lack of pleasure in daily activities), **alogia** (unwillingness to speak), and loss of libido (sex drive). These negative symptoms occur in some patients with PD, as well as some patients with dementia, suggesting a possible link.

Depression and deep brain stimulation. Recent studies with deep brain stimulation (DBS—discussed later) in people with PD are beginning to outline an anatomy of depression that complements the chemistry of depression. Some patients who receive DBS may become acutely depressed or experience mania with no apparent reason, depending on the location of the stimulator. The depression or mania subsides when the

Anergia

Lack of physical and mental energy.

Anhedonia

Lack of pleasure in daily activities.

Alogia

Unwillingness to speak.

stimulator is turned off. Stimulation near the substantia nigra and subthalamic nucleus may excite or inhibit a system of dopamine or serotonin neurons in the mesocortical and mesolimbic regions.

It is assumed that the depression of PD patients resembles that of non-PD patients, but this may be incorrect. There is evidence that depression is an integral part of PD, implying a specific biochemical and structural basis for the depression of PD, yet currently there are no specific drugs for treating the depression of PD.

Treatment of depression starts with a frank discussion between you and your family about why you're depressed. The discussion should then involve your doctor. Treatment may consist of counseling, behavior modification, or psychiatric analysis. Antidepressant drugs may be prescribed.

There are several classes of antidepressant drugs and specific reasons for using one class over another. The reasons that lead doctors to choose one class over another include the presence of anxiety, agitation or psychosis, apathy and other "negative" symptoms, rapid cycling, and dementia. The dose of a particular drug in a particular class will vary depending on age (older people don't tolerate the same dose as younger people), and the presence of dementia.

Tricyclic antidepressants (TCAs) are older drugs. There are several TCAs and each of them has varying degrees of ability to block the reuptake and raise the level of the major chemical messengers that mediate depression. Some of the TCAs are soporific—they promote sleep—and some have anti-anxiety as well as

Tricyclic antidepressants

Tricyclic antidepressants are medicines that relieve mental depression.

antidepressant activity. Some of the TCAs even have analgesic effects—they decrease pain. But all of the TCAs have varying degrees of anticholinergic activity, and this is responsible for most of their side effects: blurred vision, dry mouth, constipation, urinary retention, cardiac arrhythmias, confusion, and memory loss. The symptoms are reversible upon stopping the drug but, nonetheless, TCAs are seldom used as antidepressants because of their side effect profile.

Selective serotonin reuptake inhibitors

The most commonly prescribed antidepressant drugs; they help both anxiety and depression.

The **selective serotonin reuptake inhibitors** (SSRIs), such as Celexa, Paxil, Prozac, and Zoloft, are the most commonly prescribed antidepressant drugs because they help both anxiety and depression. They raise the levels of serotonin in the brain, and low levels of serotonin are associated with depression and anxiety. SSRIs don't cause drowsiness, which is important in PD patients who are drowsy. The SSRIs have fewer side effects than TCAs, which is why they're so widely prescribed. SSRIs take at least 2 to 3 weeks to work. Side effects include fatigue, weight gain, and loss of libido. Wellbutrin increases brain dopamine levels in all regions of the brain, not just the ones PD impacts, and is helpful in the apathetic depression of PD. Side effects include agitation and, rarely, seizures. If a patient does not improve on one SSRI, it's worthwhile to try a second SSRI.

Selective norepinephrine reuptake inhibitors

Antidepressant drugs which increase brain levels of norepinephrine, not serotonin.

Selective norepinephrine reuptake inhibitors (SNRIs) increase brain levels of norepinephrine, not serotonin. The SNRIs appear more useful in patients who are apathetic, anergic, anhedonic, and who suffer from chronic pain. Their side effect profile is similar to that of the SSRIs with the exception of possibly increased cardiac side effects. If a patient fails on SSRIs, a trial of an SNRI is reasonable. The SNRIs include Cymbalta,

Effexor, and Wellbutrin. Wellbutrin has a mild anti-Parkinson effect because it increases dopamine in the brain.

If agitation or psychosis (delusions, hallucinations, and paranoia) are significant components of the depression, an underlying cause for the agitation or psychosis should be sought. Such causes include dehydration, infections, anticholinergic and stimulant drugs (amphetamines, Ritalin). If no underlying cause is found, an SSRI combined with a tranquillizer such as quetiapine (Seroquel) might be helpful. If anxiety is a significant component, an SSRI or SNRI is a good first choice. If negative symptoms are prominent components of the depression, it is important to determine whether the patient is evolving a dementia. A few patients with severe depression, negative symptoms, are unresponsive to antidepressants, and are not demented, may respond to electric shock. In the past, this treatment has had a bad reputation, but modern electric shock is different than that used in the past and should be a treatment consideration.

If agitation or psychosis (delusions, hallucinations, and paranoia) are significant components of the depression, an underlying cause for the agitation or psychosis should be sought.

73. What are the symptoms of psychosis?

The following questions and answers highlight some of the mental changes that occur in PD.

Question 1: My father is 55 years old and has had PD for 5 years. Recently, he was started on amantadine. He's now hallucinating: he sees his father who's barking at him like a dog. Is my father demented?

Answer 1: 55 years of age is "old enough for PD" but too young for PD dementia (also called Lewy Body Dementia [LBD]). Amantadine has anticholinergic properties and can cause hallucinations.

The hallucinations are consistent with a drug-induced psychosis as well as LBD. PD dementia, like PD itself, evolves slowly over time. Your father's psychosis seems clearly precipitated by amantadine and, thus, is reversible. It should end within several days of stopping amantadine.

Question 2: My father is 80 years old. Previously, he had been an investment banker. He has had PD for 10 years and has been on levodopa/carbidopa for 8 years. In the past two years, he has started to sleep during the day, has stopped paying attention to his investments, and has difficulty remembering the names of his grandchildren. Six months ago, he began having trouble controlling his urine. Two weeks ago, he started Ditropan. Yesterday, he accused my mother, who is 78 years old, of having an affair with his brother, who is 85 years old. He also accused my mother and his brother of planning to steal his money and place him in a nursing home. Is my father demented?

Answer 2: Your father shows all the signs of evolving a dementia. Symptoms of dementia include daytime drowsiness, apathy, loss of interest, an inability to understand things which once were understandable, and memory loss. In addition to having a dementia, your father has developed a psychosis. Symptoms of psychosis in your father include delusions (a belief in something with no basis in reality) and paranoia (belief that people are seeking to do him harm). In your father, the psychosis was precipitated by Ditropan. Ditropan and other drugs which regulate the bladder are anticholinergic—they block acetylcholine, which is a necessary chemical in the brain. Older people, and especially people who are evolving a dementia, are more sensitive to anticholinergic drugs. Stop Ditropan and your father's delusions and paranoia (but not dementia) will stop.

Question 3: My 55-year-old mother was diagnosed with PD 5 years ago and was started on a dopamine agonist. Six months ago, levodopa/carbidopa was added. Yesterday, my father told me my mother had lost all of her savings through gambling. She had never gambled in her life, yet now she has become a compulsive gambler. Is this part of PD?

Answer 3: Obsessions are thoughts you cannot get out of your head and compulsions are acts which you cannot stop yourself from performing. Some PD patients on PD drugs (agonists, Sinemet) develop obsessions and compulsions. These may include obsessions with cleanliness, germs, or with dying. Compulsions may be to shop, gamble, or talk incessantly. Obsessions and compulsions are more common than thought, but people who have them may not report them until they're in trouble. For your mother, decreasing her drugs, counseling, and supervision are needed.

Question 4: My mother is 60 years old and divorced from my father. She was diagnosed with the "non-trembling" type of PD two years ago. She is a very successful literary agent. She takes levodopa/carbidopa three times a day, but a week ago she had her gall bladder removed and her levodopa was stopped. The surgery was longer and more difficult than expected. When she awoke from anesthesia she was perfectly alert and asked the doctors detailed and incisive questions about her surgery. She was in the ICU for three days and during this time she did not receive her Sinemet. On the third day, she began to eat and levodopa was re-started. As she was about to leave the

ICU, she saw a "giant white rat," became anxious, shook uncontrollably, forgot where she was, and shouted obscenities. Is she psychotic or delirious? Is this related to levodopa withdrawal?

Answer 4: Your mother was mentally sharp with no evidence of dementia or psychosis before entering the hospital. She was well immediately after surgery, so a complication of the surgery or anesthesia is not responsible. She is on a small enough dose of levodopa that stopping even for 3 days should not cause her to become psychotic or delirious. Additionally, stopping levodopa should not cause her to tremble uncontrollably, especially when tremor was not part of her PD. Unless she has a fever or severe derangement in her electrolytes, something other than PD or stopping her levodopa precipitated her behavior. One difficult scenario to consider is: could your mother be an alcoholic? For people who live alone, the scope and extent of their drinking is often not suspected until others enter their homes. In this situation, the three days your mother was in the hospital were three days in which she was withdrawing from alcohol, which precipitated alcoholic withdrawal tremors ("DTs"). This emphasizes how important it is to look for causes of psychosis other than drugs for PD.

Lewy body dementia (LBD) occurs before PD is diagnosed. Some experts regard PD dementia and LBD as different, others regard them as identical.

74. What is Lewy body dementia?

PD dementia occurs in patients who were diagnosed with PD at least one year before they were diagnosed with dementia. Lewy body dementia (LBD) occurs before PD is diagnosed. Some experts regard PD dementia and LBD as different, others regard them as identical. The pathology is similar: the loss of cells in cortical and subcortical regions and the presence of alpha-synuclein and Lewy bodies. As a general rule, though, there is a 10- to 20-year "lag" between the development of PD and the development of LBD.

LBD is slowly progressive, like PD. Likewise, the cause of dementia, like the cause of PD, is unknown. In PD, the loss of cells starts in a region called the dorsal vagal nucleus, part of the parasympathetic nervous system (the "calming center"). From there, the loss of cells goes on to affect a series of other sites in the brain that regulate alertness, sleep, behavior, thinking, balance, movement, and emotions. Next the loss of cells affects the substantia nigra.

The loss of neurons in LBD follows a similar process, starting in the dorsal vagal nucleus and moving on from there to other areas of the brain. Patients with LBD, however, also show a loss of neurons in the amygdala, which regulates anxiety. The amygdala receives images and sounds, relays them to the hippocampus (a memory bank) which compares arriving images and sounds with stored images and sounds, and tells the person if these images are dangerous, hostile, and threatening, or safe, friendly, and pleasant. In dementia and psychosis, the connections of the amygdala to the hippocampus are deranged. Friendly, pleasant images and sounds are distorted, becoming hostile and threatening. Or images and sounds stored in the hippocampus, but not present in the outside environment, are projected onto the cortex as visual or auditory hallucinations. These distortions are incredibly distressing to patients who cannot always separate them from reality.

Distinguishing LBD from Other Dementias: Depending upon the specific region affected, and the extent and degree to which it is affected, a variety of behavioral, cognitive, language, mood, memory, sleep-related and psychiatric symptoms may appear. The type and variety of symptoms vary from person to person. Although there's overlap, the time of appearance, the degree of severity, and the type and variety of symptoms often allows one dementia to be distinguished from another. Other diseases your doctor may consider in making an accurate diagnosis are: Alzheimer's disease (AD), fronto-temporal dementia (Pick's disease), vascular dementia, neurosyphilis, depression with psychotic features, and side-effects of medication.

75. What is the difference between dementia and psychosis?

Lewy body dementia has *negative symptoms* that result from a loss of dopamine, norepinephrine, serotonin, and acetylcholine cells in different brain regions. These symptoms include difficulty in calculating, concentrating, finding words, orientating, recognizing, remembering, and thinking. The psychosis consists of *positive symptoms*, which may include acting-out or aggression, delusions, hallucinations, and paranoia.

Although a psychosis may uncover or "unmask" an underlying dementia, psychosis does not necessarily mean a person has a dementia or will develop a dementia. A psychosis is reversible if the cause is found, while dementia is not reversible. The PD psychosis resembles the psychosis in young people, without dementia, who overdose on drugs such as amphetamine, methamphetamine, cocaine, and ecstasy. The psychosis resembles, in part, the psychosis of schizophrenia. The following psychoses are often encountered:

ICU psychosis: In this case a patient in an ICU, where bells are ringing, beepers beeping, lights flashing, and strangers coming and going, becomes sleep deprived and develops a psychosis. There may or may not be an underlying dementia.

Post-operative psychosis: A patient may develop a psychosis related to the type and duration of surgery and anesthesia, the severity of blood loss, and the type and amount of fluids administered during the operation. There may or may not be an underlying dementia.

"Sundowning" psychosis: A patient who is in strange surroundings (often in nursing care facilities) may develop a psychosis at night. There is usually an underlying dementia.

Delirium tremens: Psychosis due to the abrupt withdrawal from alcohol. Other causes include dehydration, fever, hypoglycemia, and kidney or liver failure.

The following contrasts the symptoms of dementia and psychosis:

Lack of Awareness. In dementia, a person does not realize or recognize that anything is wrong. This results, in part, from changes in the right cerebral hemisphere. In psychosis, a person is hyper-aware of his surroundings. He may have illusions: transforming one object into another; hallucinations: seeing objects and people who aren't present or are dead; or delusions and paranoia: imagining people are trying to harm him. Hyper-awareness is one of the main distinctions between psychosis and dementia.

Lack of Alertness. In dementia, the person seems to "sleep" all day. This results, in part, from changes in the sleep centers in the brainstem. These centers are near the substantia nigra and the locus ceruleus. In psychosis, the person is awake all night. He may or may not sleep during the day.

Difficulty with memory. This is apparent in dementia and results from loss of cells in the hippocampus and temporal lobes. In psychosis, a person's memory may be intact, but he may be so anxious or so distracted he "can't remember" or won't let himself be tested.

Difficulty paying attention. A person may have a short attention span in both dementia and psychosis, but for different reasons. For instance, a person with dementia can't remember how to spell a word such as W-O-R-L-D backward, while a person with psychosis can't pay attention long enough to spell W-O-R-L-D backward. In both cases, the person may be easily distracted.

Disorientation. In dementia, the person may not know the day or month or that a major event has occurred (such as destruction of the World Trade Center). He may not know where he is and may become confused in a new place. If a person with psychosis can be made to pay attention and be tested, he will be oriented, at least to place.

Difficulty with spatial relationships. People with either dementia or psychosis may be unable to follow directions or instructions. They may be unable to organize, plan, or think of new ideas, though this may be for different reasons. This results from changes in the frontal lobes.

Restricted mood. A person with dementia is apathetic; he takes no interest in people or his surroundings. He appears depressed but he's not, as he lacks the main features of depression: sadness, guilt, and feeling ashamed. In psychosis, a person's moods are inappropriate: he's happy when others are sad. The person's moods are boisterous, upbeat, but changing: he goes from being "down" to "up" to "down" for no apparent reason. In his "up" moods, he's inappropriate and unreasonable, may be excessively anxious, and may panic easily.

Obsessions and Compulsions. In dementia, a person may have "passive" compulsions: he may hum or repeat stereotyped phrases over and over, like a parrot. In psychosis, a person may have "active but destructive" obsessions and compulsions. He may be obsessed with cleanliness or germs to the exclusion of all activities. He may have a compulsion to gamble, collect trash, or engage in aberrant sexual behavior: cross-dressing, pornography, prostitution.

The psychosis associated with LBD: delusions, hallucinations, paranoia, agitation, and acting-out, are what leads to nursing home placement. The care-partner or family of the person with PD and motor disability may have been able to deal with the patient's physical disability, but are unable to deal with the psychotic behavior. The psychosis resembles the psychosis of schizophrenia; consequently, drugs used in schizophrenia that block dopamine receptors (neuroleptics) are used to treat the psychosis of LBD. Although it's unclear if similar mechanisms are involved, neuroleptics have become the mainstay of treatment. The traditional neuroleptics such as Haldol and Thorazine aggravate PD, and this has led to the use of atypical neuroleptics such as Quetiapine or Seroquel. Seroquel is sedating, and thus is helpful to agitated patients who have difficulty falling asleep.

The psychosis associated with LBD: delusions, hallucinations, paranoia, agitation, and acting-out, are what leads to nursing home placement.

189

Reports of unexplained deaths in elderly patients taking neuroleptics, including Seroquel, have resulted in a "black box warning" appearing on the package. Whether those deaths are drug-related or coincidental is unclear. Elderly patients who are demented and psychotic may die for reasons unrelated to their use of a neuroleptic. The "black box warning" has created caution in prescribing neuroleptics and, at present, they are reserved for truly intolerable behavior: screaming, punching or kicking the care-partner, or constantly calling the police. Abilify, or aripiprazole, is another atypical neuroleptic. Clozaril remains the "gold standard" of anti-psychotic drugs but requires weekly blood counts and periodic cardiac evaluations. Clozaril is reserved for patients who've failed on Seroquel and Abilify.

Zofran, an anti-emetic drug that blocks serotonin receptors in the brain, is occasionally used to treat psychotic behavior. The drug was introduced by Dr. Eldad Melamed as a non-dopamine receptor blocker. The basis for believing serotonin plays a role in psychosis is the observation that LSD and ecstasy—drugs that induce delusions, hallucinations and paranoia—do so by increasing brain serotonin levels. Pimavanserin is a drug, currently being investigated, that may block the development of hallucinations and delusions more effectively than Zofran.

The dementia of LBD, like the dementia of Alzheimer's disease, is associated with a loss of acetylcholine neurons in several regions of the brain. The nucleus basalis, a region at the base of the globus pallidus, is a rich source of acetylcholine neurons, and is affected early in LBD and Alzheimer's disease. The nucleus basalis has rich connections to the amygdala, the hippocampus, and the cingulate gyrus, regions of the brain that mediate behavior, emotion, and alertness. Treatment of LBD and Alzheimer's disease uses cholinesterase inhibitors, which block the enzyme cholinesterase that breaks down acetylcholine. This increases the concentration of acetylcholine near muscarine and nicotine receptors. Three cholinesterase inhibitors are available: rivastigmine or Exelon, donepezil or Aricept, and galantamine or Razadyne. These drugs cross the blood brain barrier and block cholinesterase in the brain, relieving many of the symptoms of LBD and Alzheimer's disease. They also delay the disability of LBD and Alzheimer's disease, allowing patients to remain at home longer. Only rivastigmine, or Exelon, is approved for the treatment of LBD. Exelon is a relatively short-acting drug that must be given orally twice a day, with a side effect of nausea at high doses. Exelon also comes in a patch. Side effects of the patch include drooling and diarrhea, but it is better tolerated and has less nausea associated with its use. Finally, memantine, or Namenda, is a drug related to amantadine. Like amantadine, Namenda blocks glutamate at the NMDA glutamate receptor, but does not have anticholinergic activity and does not causes confusion, delusions, or memory loss. Namenda is approved as a second-line drug for treating Alzheimer's disease and, while it is not approved for LBD, it is sometimes helpful when added to Exelon.

PART SIX

What Else Should I Know?

What is deep brain stimulation?

What is the role of gene therapy in Parkinson disease treatment?

How can I make my home safer?

When will there be a cure?

More...

76. What is deep brain stimulation?

Stimulation surgery, or deep brain stimulation (DBS) refers to implanting a probe or electrode (a stimulator) into a clearly defined, abnormally discharging brain region—a region generating "static"—the subthalamic nucleus, the globus pallidus, or the thalamus (which one requires an expert opinion). By generating a blocking or inhibiting counter-current, the effects of the static are lessened or negated. Technically, DBS is a misnomer—the abnormally discharging brain region isn't stimulated; rather it is blocked or inhibited by a reverse counter-current that "turns off" the abnormal "static" in the region.

There is renewed interest in DBS because it is seen as a refinement of thalamotomy and pallidotomy.

There is renewed interest in DBS because it is seen as a refinement of thalamotomy and pallidotomy. However, instead of destroying a section of brain tissue, DBS uses a high-frequency electrical charge to stimulate the brain. Where the electrode is placed in the brain determines which symptoms will be alleviated. During surgery, a micro-electrode is permanently implanted in a specific region. Wires from the implanted electrode are then passed beneath the skin (where they are invisible) to a small battery pack placed under the skin near the shoulder. This device is then adjusted to the patient's own needs, to regulate the frequency of the electrode. The patient will be able to turn it off and on by means of a magnet. When the device is on, the stimulation will stop the tremor, the dyskinesia, or improve the bradykinesia within a few seconds. When it is turned off, the tremor or dyskinesia will return.

The major advantage of this surgery is that it has fewer complications than thalamotomy or pallidotomy and there is significant improvement of symptoms, sometimes requiring smaller amounts of PD drugs. The regions targeted by DBS are the thalamus, the globus pallidus, and the subthalamic nucleus. Increasingly, the subthalamic nucleus is becoming the preferred target. The subthalamic nucleus is located below the thalamus, and it acts as a "brake" on the substantia nigra. DBS can be a treatment option for PD patients who are no longer responding satisfactorily to their PD medications, or for those who have developed dykinesias. DBS can help to reduce or eliminate tremor and dystonia.

Studies have compared DBS to thalamotomy and pallidotomy and, although sufficient data still need to be collected, these studies have shown much more results in favor of DBS. How long does DBS last? It is difficult to tell. The best answer is that DBS holds certain symptoms, such as tremor and dyskinesia in check; unfortunately, other symptoms, such as difficulty walking, difficulty with balance, difficulty with thinking and memory, progress at the rate they would have progressed had you not had DBS.

DBS is painless. The scalp, which contains pain-sensitive nerves, is numbed with a local anesthetic. Next, a small hole is drilled into the skull. The skull and underlying brain covering, the dura, contain pain-sensitive nerves, so they are also numbed with a local anesthetic. The brain itself contains no pain-sensitive nerves.

Whether DBS is done on one side of the brain or both varies from institution to institution. At the Barrow Neurological Institute, DBS is done on the side of the brain opposite the side of the body with the worse symptoms. Your right thalamus, globus pallidus, and subthalamic nucleus control symptoms on the left side of your body, and vice versa. About one or two weeks after the initial surgery, a judgment is made as to whether surgery should be done on the opposite side of the brain. Most patients with PD need surgery on both sides of the brain because by the time they seek surgery, their symptoms involve both sides of their body. Some institutions stage the surgery: one operation followed several days or weeks later by a second operation, while some institutions do both operations at the same time.

It's estimated there are 1,000,000 PD patients in the United States, and fewer than 5,000 patients (0.5% of PD patients) undergo DBS each year. Fewer patients opt for this treatment because the surgery isn't for newly diagnosed patients, patients doing well on drugs, patients with advanced disease who aren't responding to drugs, those with hallucinations, confusion, or memory loss, or patients who are hesitant or afraid.

DBS is a surgical treatment, and any surgery, even when done at a world-class institution such as the Barrow Neurological Institute, carries a risk. DBS carries a risk of 1% (one in a hundred) to 3% of stroke or hemorrhage in the brain. At the BNI, where the surgeons are experienced and where almost 100 DBS procedures are done annually, there is at least a 1% of risk of stroke or hemorrhage. Additional risks include infection. The risk is higher if both sides of the brain are operated upon. With bilateral DBS, a few patients note a decrease in the volume of their voices, a few note more difficulty with their balance, and a few become depressed. All risks and consequences are explained by a surgeon prior to the procedure.

77. Who is not a candidate for DBS?

People who have disorders that resemble PD, so-called PD-plus disorders or PD-like disorders, but who have *not* responded to levodopa, are not candidates for

DBS. Prior to being considered for DBS, all PD patients will undergo an evaluation in which their levodopa is stopped for 16 hours. then examined, followed by a test dose of levodopa and another examination after the levodopa has had a chance to work. Only patients in whom levodopa is still working, although working erratically, will be considered for DBS.

To determine your candidacy for DBS, your doctor will conduct an evaluation that consists of taking a history and examining you to determine if you are a candidate for DBS. If you are, the specialist will make a second appointment for you, during which you will be evaluated while off your medicine for 16 hours, and again after you have taken your medicine. You will then be referred to a neuropsychologist and will have an MRI. The evaluation is usually completed in one day. Following the evaluation, an appointment will be arranged with the neurosurgeon.

Perhaps only 10% of PD patients are candidates for surgery. As surgery is improved and perfected, as it becomes safer and new techniques and strategies are innovated, developed, and applied, a larger number of patients may opt for and benefit from surgery.

78. What is lesion or ablative surgery?

Ablative, or destructive, surgery refers to locating, targeting, then ablating or destroying a specific, clearly defined brain area or region—one that has been altered or changed by PD. Ablative surgery targets a region that generates an abnormal chemical or electrical discharge, which in turn generates an abnormal signal or "static." The static, in turn, interrupts the normal, harmonious operation of the brain. Destruction of the

Ablative surgery targets a region that generates an abnormal chemical or electrical discharge, which in turn generates an abnormal signal or "static."

abnormally discharging brain region lessens or negates the static and allows restoration of more normal or closer-to-normal function. However, destruction of the abnormally discharging region rarely results in restoration of completely normal function.

Why doesn't destruction of the abnormally discharging region restore normal function? The brain is more than a circuit board. There's more wrong in PD than one abnormally discharging region. Only part of the abnormally discharging region may have been destroyed and, at a later date, the surgeon may have to re-operate. To understand why only part of the abnormally discharging region may be destroyed requires understanding of the surgical procedure.

To ablate or destroy the abnormal discharging region, the surgeon heats the exploring probe or electrode—this coagulates, denatures, and destroys the abnormal region. Because the patient is awake during surgery, the surgeon can monitor the extent of the ablation by observing the patient's response. As an example, a patient with a left-hand tremor has the probe inserted into his brain's right-side. The brain's right-side controls the body's left-side and vice-versa. The surgeon then heats, coagulates, and destroys part of the patient's right thalamus, the abnormally discharging region. The abnormal electrical discharge is monitored through the probe—the same probe that later heats, coagulates, and destroys the abnormal region. When the patient's tremor ceases, the probe is removed. Heating causes the surrounding thalamus to swell. Initially, the heat-induced swelling inactivates a wider region than is required to stop the tremor. After several days or weeks, the heat-induced swelling subsides. Part of the thalamus remains quiet, no longer discharging. But part may recover and the tremor may return. Few surgeons can correctly estimate the size and intensity of the burn needed to permanently abolish a tremor. It's safer to induce a smaller burn, to destroy a smaller region, and chance the tremor returning then to destroy a larger region and risk paralysis. This is why the results of DBS, in which tissue is not destroyed, are generally thought better than those of ablative surgery.

79. What is deep brain stimulation of the subthalamic nucleus?

The subthalamic nucleus (STN), or subthalamus, is a region of your brain below the thalamus and near the substantia nigra. If your STN is destroyed by a stroke or tumor, you develop violent involuntary movements on the opposite side of your body. The movements, called hemiballismus, resemble someone repeatedly throwing a shot-put, or hurling a discus. The STN normally acts as a "brake" on your substantia nigra. If you think of your brain as a car, your substantia nigra acts like your accelerator. In PD, your nigra (accelerator) slows down and your STN (brake) is "released" instead of being turned off. Thus you slow down for two reasons: your accelerator's not working and your brake is on. When you're treated with levodopa, your accelerator "speeds up" and your brake is released, and you may develop dyskinesia, a cousin of hemiballismus. Initially surgeons were reluctant to place an electrode in the STN because they were afraid to cause hemiballismus. Dr. A. Benemid showed that DBS of the STN not only improved bradykinesia by partially releasing the brake on the substantia nigra, but that DBS of the STN also decreased dyskinesia and tremor. DBS of the STN is now the most widely used procedure for treating PD because the results are more consistent than DBS of the globus pallidus. The exception

DBS of the STN is now the most widely used procedure for treating PD because the results are more consistent than DBS of the globus pallidus.

is dystonia; this symptom responds best to DBS of the globus pallidus.

One of the many future roles of DBS will be to develop new targets; regions of the brain that modulate walking and balance, anxiety and depression, mood swings and compulsions. Thus, the prepontine nucleus (PPN), a region of the brain below the substantia nigra that projects upward to the cortex and downward to the spinal cord, is affected in PD and in some of the PD-like disorders such as progressive supranuclear palsy (PSP) and corticobasilar degeneration (CBD). Preliminary studies of DBS of the PPN suggest that it may improve freezing of gait and the difficulty with balance that accompanies advanced PD, PSP, and CBD.

80. What about transplantation?

Restorative, or transplantation, surgery implants dopamine-producing cells into the striatum. In the striatum (which is composed of the caudate nucleus and the putamen) fibers project downward from the cerebral cortex, co-mingling with dopamine fibers that project upward from the substantia nigra. Cells are transplanted into the striatum because it's easier and safer to locate and target than the smaller and less accessible substantia nigra. Because the foreign cells aren't transplanted into the nigra, they can't exactly replicate the function of the lost neurons in the nigra. As an example, dopamine neurons in the nigra receive, exchange, analyze, process, and interpret information from other brain regions including serotonin neurons in the brain stem (a region below the nigra) and the subthalamic nucleus. Dopamine neurons transplanted into the striatum don't receive, exchange, analyze, process, and interpret information from the brain stem or STN.

Transplanted cells can come from several sources: your adrenal gland, your carotid arteries, human or pig embryos, or stem cells. Once implanted, the cells then attempt to compensate for the lost neurons in your substantia nigra. Approximately 80–90% of transplanted cells die during transplantation, failing to take hold or establish connections within the patient's brain. Successful transplantation usually requires at least 1,600,000 cells. Restorative surgery seeks to re-establish dopamine levels in your brain while setting back the "PD clock"—returning you to a less advanced disease stage.

Successful transplantation usually requires at least 1,600,000 cells.

Transplantation is usually performed bilaterally. In some hospitals, surgery is performed on both sides in the same setting; however, other hospitals choose to perform the surgery in stages: first one side, then several weeks or months later, the other side. The surgery is performed stereotaxically, meaning the patient is asleep. The surgery carries approximately the same risks as ablative surgery: a 1% to 3% risk of hemorrhage, stroke, or death. Unlike ablative surgery or DBS, the benefits of transplantation aren't apparent for months because the transplanted cells must establish and integrate themselves into your brain. Most, but not all, patients who undergo transplantation surgery are treated with immunosuppressive drugs to prevent the brain from rejecting the cells. A research study demonstrated that transplantation is moderately beneficial in some patients, predominantly those less than 60 years old. However, many of these patients developed dyskinesia and, in some patients, the dyskinesias were so bothersome as to require DBS of the STN. Long term follow-up revealed that most patients, after an initial improvement, showed progression of their PD.

81. What is the role of stem cells in Parkinson disease treatment?

Stem cells are primitive cells that have the ability to divide countless times and to transform themselves into specialized cells. Life begins when a sperm fertilizes an egg and creates a single cell that has the potential to be a human being. This fertilized egg is called totipotent because it can generate every cell in the body. This is an embryonic stem cell. In the first hours after fertilization, this cell divides into identical totipotent cells. If either of these cells is placed into a woman's uterus, either cell can develop into a human being. In fact, identical twins develop when two totipotent cells separate and develop into two genetically identical human beings.

Four days after fertilization and after several cycles of cell division, these totipotent cells specialize, forming a hollow sphere called a blastocyst. The cyst has an outer and an inner layer of cells. The outer cells will form the placenta. The inner cells will form all the tissues of the human body. Although the inner cells form almost every type of human cell, they cannot form a human being. These inner cells are called pluripotent and are also embryonic stem cells but, because they are not totipotent, they are not embryos. If the inner cells were placed into a woman's uterus, they would not develop into a human being. The pluripotent cells undergo specialization into stem cells that subsequently give rise to cells that have a particular function. Examples of these stem cells include blood stem cells which give rise to red blood cells, white blood cells and platelets; skin stem cells that give rise to the various types of skin cells. These stem cells are called multipotent and are present in both children and adults. Thus, blood stem cells exist in the bone marrow of everyone and you cannot survive without them.

A technique called somatic cell nuclear transfer (SCNT) is a way of isolating pluripotent stem cells. Using SCNT, researchers take a normal animal egg cell and remove the nucleus (the structure containing the chromosomes). The material left behind in the egg contains nutrients that are essential for embryo development. Then, any cell other than an egg or a sperm cell is placed next to the egg from which the nucleus has been removed, and the two are fused. The resulting fused cell and its immediate descendants are totipotent: they have the potential to develop into an entire animal. These totipotent cells will form a blastocyst. Cells from the inner cells of the blastocyst could, in theory, be used to develop pluripotent stem cell lines.

At the most fundamental level, pluripotent stem cells can help us understand the events that occur during human development. A goal of this work is the identification of the factors involved in the decision-making process that results in cell specialization. We know that turning genes on and off is central to this process, but we do not know much about these "decision-making" genes or what turns them on or off. Some of our most serious medical conditions, such as cancer and birth defects, are due to abnormal cell specialization and cell division. A better understanding of normal cell processes may allow us to correct these conditions.

Some of our most serious medical conditions, such as cancer and birth defects, are due to abnormal cell specialization and cell division.

Human pluripotent stem cell research may dramatically change the way we develop drugs and test them for safety. For example, new drugs could be initially tested using human cell lines. Cell lines are currently used in this way (for example, cancer cells). Pluripotent stem cells would allow testing in more cell types and this would streamline the process of drug development. Only the drugs that are both safe and effective in cell line testing would graduate to further testing in laboratory animals and human subjects. The most far-reaching potential of human pluripotent stem cells is the generation of cells and tissue that could be used in "cell therapies." Many diseases result from disruption of cellular function or destruction of tissues. Today, donated organs and tissues are often used to replace ailing organs. However, the number of people suffering from these disorders outstrips the number of organs available for transplantation. Pluripotent stem cells, stimulated to develop into specialized cells, offer the possibility of a renewable source of replacement cells and tissue to treat PD, Alzheimer's disease, spinal cord injury, stroke, burns, heart disease, diabetes, and arthritis.

Several laboratories have developed dopamine-producing neurons from adult stem cells. The idea is to use these neurons to replace the dead or dying neurons in the substantia nigra of PD patients. One limitation in this approach is that PD is more than a loss of neurons in the nigra, and replacing the missing neurons will correct some, but not all, of the symptoms of PD. A second limitation is that the cells will not halt the progression of PD. However, it is possible that, in the future, dopamine neurons made from adult stem cells will prove beneficial in PD.

82. What are growth or trophic factors?

Hormones are chemical messengers secreted into the blood by glands to regulate activities of vital organs. The best known hormone is insulin, produced in the pancreas. When production of insulin declines or ceases, diabetes results. Insulin is considered a growth factor because it nourishes or sustains cells.

Human growth hormone (HGH), secreted by the pituitary gland, is a small protein-like hormone (peptide), similar to insulin. It is secreted in brief pulses during the early hours of sleep and remains in circulation for only a few minutes. It's quickly bound to HGH receptors throughout the body. With the development of recombinant DNA technology, HGH and glial-derived neurotrophic factor (GDNF)—a hormone or growth factor secreted by the support cells of the brain, are available in pure form.

Approximately every three years, 90% of the cells in your body are made anew. Only the original cells (neurons) in the brain are retained for many years. But even in the brain, new cells, proteins, and growth factors are continuously being produced. Learning, memory, intelligence, movement, and balance all depend on growth factors. As growth factors such as HGH and GDNF fall with age, functions of all tissues, including the dopamine cells in the substantia nigra, decrease. The dopamine cells in the substantia nigra are stimulated by GDNF.

Approximately every three years, 90% of the cells in your body are made anew.

The reason the regulation of HGH, like GDNF and other growth factors, is complex is that, if unregulated, these factors could produce mutations or cancers. In PD, GDNF is required to nourish and sustain dopamine neurons. In the absence of GDNF, the dopamine neurons die. Several attempts have been made to deliver GDNF directly to these dying neurons in the substantia nigra. Because GDNF is a peptide, it cannot be given by mouth because it is broken down in the stomach. It also cannot be given by injection because it doesn't cross the blood-brain barrier. Initially, GDNF was infused into the spinal fluid; however it didn't reach the neurons in the substantia nigra in sufficiently high quantities to be effective. Next, GDNF was infused through a catheter directly into the substantia nigra. In a study conducted several years ago, there was a debate as to the effectiveness of the treatment. Some investigators claimed substantial improvement, others didn't. The limitation of the study is that the infusion of GDNF does not replicate the manner in which naturally-produced GDNF is regulated and taken up into the nigra. To overcome these limitations, the DNA for several GDNF-like growth factors were cloned, multiplied, and inserted into a virus. The virus was then delivered into different regions in the brain, invaded the neurons in these regions, transferred the growth factor DNA to the neurons, and made the neurons manufacture and secrete enough of the growth factor to repair themselves.

83. What is the role of gene therapy in Parkinson disease treatment?

In gene therapy a carrier, called a vector, is used to deliver a gene into target cells of a patient. Currently, the most common vectors are viruses that have been genetically engineered to carry human DNA. Viruses have evolved a way of packaging and delivering their genes into human cells and doctors are trying to harness this ability. In PD, target neurons such as those in the substantia nigra and the subthalamic nucleus are infected with the virus, which then unloads its genetic material containing the gene into the target neuron. The generation of a growth factor or an enzyme from the inserted gene helps restore the target neuron to a normal state.

All viruses attack their hosts and introduce their genetic material into the host cells as part of their replication cycle. This genetic material contains basic 'instructions' of how to produce more copies of the virus, hijacking the cells' normal production machinery to serve the needs of the virus. The host cells will carry out these instructions and produce additional copies of the virus, leading to more and more cells becoming infected. Some viruses physically insert their genes into the host's genome. This incorporates the genes of that virus among the genes of the host for the life span of the cell.

Adeno-associated viruses, AAV, are small viruses with a genome consisting of a single stranded DNA. The AAV does not integrate into the human genome. Instead, the recombinant viral genome fuses into a circular form which becomes the means through which the gene expresses itself (makes an enzyme or a growth factor). The disadvantages to using an AAV include the small amount of DNA it can carry and the difficulty in making it. AAV are currently being used by themselves because they're harmless. Two trials with an AAV in PD are ongoing.

The disadvantages of gene therapy include:

The short-lived nature of the therapy. Before gene therapy can become a permanent cure for any condition, the genetic material introduced into target cells must remain functional and the cells containing the material must be long-lived and stable. Problems with integrating viral genetic material into the genome and the rapidly dividing nature of some cells prevent gene therapy from achieving long-term benefits. Many patients may have to undergo multiple rounds of gene therapy.

The immune response. Any time a foreign object, such as a virus, is introduced into human tissues, the immune system mounts an attack on the invader. The risk of stimulating the immune system so that it decreases or abolishes the effectiveness of the therapy is a possibility.

84. How safe is anesthesia for people with Parkinson disease?

Every day, people with PD, like people without PD, face surgery. This includes relatively minor surgeries such as tooth extraction, biopsy of a mole, biopsy of a breast, colonoscopy, or cataract surgery, as well as major surgeries such as coronary artery bypass, removal of a cancerous lung, repair of a ruptured aneurysm, or surgery on the back or neck for a herniated disc and/or spinal stenosis. In addition, people with PD are more likely than people without PD to undergo surgery for a broken hip or shoulder (as a result of a fall) or deep brain stimulation (DBS).

Modern day anesthesia and surgery are relatively safe and patients who, in the recent past, were "too sick" to have surgery because of failing hearts or lungs, or advanced age, are now able to undergo surgery.

Surgery, although painless because of anesthesia, places major physical and psychological stresses on a person. These are the psychological stresses of anticipation, fear, and uncertainty. Thus, if the surgery is for a tumor, you may worry if the tumor is benign or malignant. Can the surgeon remove all of the tumor or only part of it? Will a second or third operation be necessary? Will I be in pain afterward?

Modern day anesthesia and surgery are relatively safe and patients who, in the recent past, were "too sick" to have surgery because of failing hearts or lungs, or advanced age, are now able to undergo surgery. But, because they have failing hearts or are advanced in age, they're more vulnerable to complications. In addition, the types of surgery being done today—deep brain stimulation, removal of formerly "inoperable" tumors, organ transplants, replacement of entire hips and knees—are more complicated, require sophisticated anesthesia and monitoring, and are more likely to result in complications even with the best and most experienced surgeons and anesthesiologists, and in the most advanced hospitals.

Generally, PD patients are more prone to the effects of anticipation and worry on the autonomic nervous system. Because the **autonomic nervous system (ANS)** constricts blood vessels, it can decrease blood supply to your heart. Thus, PD patients are more prone to the rises and falls of blood pressure during surgery. Older patients may become agitated or confused, delusional, disoriented, or have hallucinations after surgery. This is called an "intensive care unit (ICU) psychosis" or "sundowning." PD patients who suffer from dementia, or who have had a history of agitation, confusion, delusions, disorientation and hallucinations on PD drugs, are more vulnerable to these complications.

A special problem for PD patients who undergo major surgery under general anesthesia, especially bowel surgery, is their inability to take anti-PD drugs by mouth following the surgery. Parcopa, carbidopa/levodopa which dissolves in the mouth, may or may not be absorbed in a bowel that, in essence, is not working. In such patients, the Neupro patch, a dopamine agonist absorbed through the skin, may be helpful. Generally, PD patients who have had PD for five years and under can tolerate several days without anti-PD drugs. But PD patients who have had PD for ten years or longer cannot usually tolerate three or more days without anti-PD drugs. Patients who have had PD for 5–10 years fall between the two extremes. Following surgery, most PD patients can be restarted on anti-PD drugs within 48 hours. In those patients who cannot be

Autonomic nervous system (ANS)

The portion of the brain and nervous system that governs or regulates the body's internal environment.

re-started on anti-PD drugs by mouth, Parcopa and/or Neupro are helpful.

If you have PD and if you need surgery, it's wise to insist on a consultation with an anesthesiologist prior to your surgery. Ask the surgeon and the anesthesiologist if the procedure can be done without general anesthesia. Local anesthesia (anesthetizing a small region), regional anesthesia, spinal and epidural anesthesia do not require muscle relaxants or intubation (insertion of a tube into the trachea) and, in general, are less physically stressful (though for some patients may be more psychologically stressful) than general anesthesia. However, local, regional, spinal, and epidural anesthesia have their own potential problems. Deciding on the appropriate type of anesthesia is done by the anesthesiologist, the surgeon and the patient. The decision is made after taking a medical history and doing a thorough examination. Factors contributing to the choice of anesthesia include the patient's attitude and the effects of the anesthesia on the patient's PD.

85. Is Botox helpful in treating Parkinson disease?

Botulinum toxin (Botox) blocks the release of acetylcholine from the nerves to your muscles, resulting in paralysis. Botox binds to a specific protein on the surface of the nerve ending, forming a Botox-protein complex. This step takes 30 minutes. Next, the membrane of the nerve folds around the complex, forming a vesicle and absorbing the complex. Inside the nerve terminal, the complex is split; Botox is released and binds to and inactivates a second protein, one that's essential to releasing acetylcholine. The effects of a Botox injection last 2-6 months, depending on the muscle injected and the amount of Botox used. As long as Botox is injected into the muscle, and not a vein, the paralysis is confined to the muscle: it's not generalized.

Botox is used to treat strabismus (eye muscle spasm), hemi-facial spasm, focal dystonia (including blepharospasm—inability to open the eyes), torticollis (wry neck), spasmodic dysphonia (squeaky voice), and writer's cramp. In addition to blocking the release of acetylcholine from your nerves to your muscles, Botox blocks the release of acetylcholine from your salivary and sweat glands.

Some PD patients suffer from painful muscular cramps—dystonia. Botox may relieve dystonia conditions such as retrocollis or torticollis (see Question 22). Note that in PD, anterocollis usually results from weakness of the muscles that keep your head up, the extensor muscles of your neck, not from a downward pull of the muscles that flex your neck, so as a rule, Botox doesn't help the anterocollis of PD. Dystonia can also result in spasm of your leg muscles, causing your feet to be turned in (pigeon-toed) or turned out, like a duck's. Having one or both of your feet turned "in" or "out" can make walking difficult and may occasionally result in freezing of gait (FOG) and falls. Botox injections into the muscles that are in spasm may relieve dystonia and improve your walking. Care must be taken in injecting Botox, though, because too much can weaken the muscles and cause you to fall. Botox injected into your salivary glands can decrease drooling. Finally, Botox injected into the sweat glands under your arms or in your groin can partially decrease sweating. However, most sweating results from the merocrine sweat glands found throughout your skin, not from the apocrine sweat glands under your arms or in your groin, which Botox targets, which is why Botox can only partially decrease sweating.

86. Does Parkinson disease affect vision?

You may have excellent vision, but find that reading is difficult. In PD, the muscles of your eyes slow down and may be less able to accommodate the rapid movements that are necessary for scanning a line of print. Occasionally, you may have double vision. This condition, related to PD, may be helped by using specially-designed prisms. A second condition related to PD may involve interpretation of the images cast on the retina by the lens of your eye. The retina contains dopamine cells, and when the dopamine system is affected in PD, it may influence your eyes. A third condition may be lack of eye blinking. Your eyes may become dry and irritated because your lids do not blink enough to wash away dust, pollen, or other irritants. This condition may be helped with artificial tears.

If you have difficulty seeing, consult an **ophthalmologist**, a medical doctor who can diagnose and treat eye conditions. Remember that you are more likely to have difficulty seeing because of conditions unrelated to PD. The eye doctor will check your visual acuity for both distance (far) vision and reading (near) vision. A common condition is **Presbyopia**, where the length of your lens changes with age and, in order to read, you're forced to hold the paper farther and farther away. A second condition is **cataracts**, in which the lens of your eye becomes cloudy and it seems as though you are looking through water. A third condition is **glaucoma**, which results from an accumulation of fluid behind the eye. The fluid presses on the optic nerves and can, over time, lead to blindness. Pain often accompanies acute glaucoma. Chronic glaucoma is usually silent—that is, you may not know you have it. The anticholinergic drugs (Artane and Cogentin) used

If you have difficulty seeing, consult an ophthalmologist, a medical doctor who can diagnose and treat eye conditions.

Ophthalmologist

A physician specializing in eye disorders.

Presbyopia

A condition of the eye in which the length of the lens changes with age.

Cataracts

A condition in which the lens of the eye becomes cloudy and obscured, usually relieved with surgery.

Glaucoma

A disease of the eyes in which fluid accumulates behind the eye and presses on the optic nerves, in time leading to blindness.

in PD treatment can increase eye pressure, especially in people with narrow-angle glaucoma.

The doctor will check the pressure in your eye to determine whether you have glaucoma. Then, using an ophthalmoscope, he or she will look at your retina. The retina is the only place in the body where the arteries (as distinct from the veins) can be examined. Looking at the arteries of the eye provides a "window" into all of the arteries elsewhere. Such information is especially helpful if you have diabetes or high blood pressure, conditions that affect the arteries. Another retinal condition that can be diagnosed with an oph-thalmoscope is macular degeneration.

87. Can I black out from Parkinson disease?

Yes, people with PD can black out. It is uncommon, but it does occur. The cause of the blackout is a decrease in blood flow to the brain. This often occurs when a person with PD arises abruptly from a lying to a sitting or standing position. When you lie down, your heart and head are at the same level. It is rela-tively easy for your heart, an electrically driven pump, to pump blood to your brain through the great arteries in the neck. When you go from a lying down to a sit-ting or standing position, your head is now higher than your heart, and your heart must pump against gravity, working harder to pump blood to your brain. In order to maintain the same blood flow to your brain, your body has three options: your ANS can make your heart beat faster (inability of your heart to beat faster due to heart disease is one of the more important causes of blackouts—as distinct from being dizzy). Such an inability to beat faster may require the placement of a pacemaker, it can increase the force of your heart's contractions so your heart can pump harder, or it can increase the resistance of the great arteries in your neck so that the arteries contract. In some people with PD, the ANS is not as responsive and thus, when they stand up from a lying or sitting position, their blood pressure drops, the great arteries in their neck do not constrict, blood flow to their brain decreases, and they black out. Certain drugs, including the dopamine agonists, can exacerbate this tendency.

Blacking out while standing in one place for a long period of time (more than 30 minutes) occurs for different reasons than does blacking out while arising from a lying or sitting to a standing position. If you stand long enough in one place, blood pools in the veins and capillaries of your feet, robbing your heart of blood needed to operate efficiently. This causes a drop in blood pressure, which in turn results in decreased blood flow to the brain, and thus leads to a blackout. Even a person who is perfectly healthy can black out if he or she stands for a long period of time. The factors increasing the tendency to black out while standing are: the length of time you stand, whether the place where you are standing is very warm or hot, the presence of other factors which could result in dehydration such as a virus, and the presence of varicose veins. Varicose veins permit increased pooling of blood in the veins of the feet and legs, making less blood available for the filling chambers of the heart. If you have varicose veins, wearing elastic stockings can help prevent blackouts by "toning" the veins.

88. Should I eat more or less protein?

As PD advances and patients on levodopa experience "wearing off" and "on-off," paying attention to protein in the diet can sometimes make a difference. The reason for this is that dietary protein causes a large peak in the concentration of certain amino acids that circulate in the bloodstream an hour after meals. These amino acids share with levodopa a "carrier" that transports them across the gut wall into the bloodstream and another "carrier" that transports them across the blood-brain barrier. When blood amino acid levels are high, levodopa uptake into the brain is low. When this happens, people "turn-off" and their PD symptoms reappear.

Additional studies in PD indicate that anything that slows the speed of gastric emptying will slow the entry of levodopa into the blood and the brain. Some of the drugs used to treat PD, such as Artane and Cogentin, slow gastric emptying. However, the chief culprit is food. For this reason it's best to take levodopa on an empty stomach. Although levodopa absorption from the stomach into the bloodstream and from the bloodstream into the brain would be optimal if people ate no protein, without protein it would not be possible to maintain good nutrition. Protein, carbohydrates and fats are the main components of our diet. However, it's possible, if necessary, to modify your diet in such a way that all of your body's requirement for protein, at least 40 grams a day, can be eaten in a single, evening meal.

Anything that slows the speed of gastric emptying will slow the entry of levodopa into the blood and the brain.

When people find that a protein redistribution diet does not help with their "wearing off" or "on-off," it may be they're unaware of the protein content of their food. The foods that contain little or no protein are, for the most part, vegetables and fruits. These can be eaten in their fresh, frozen, canned, stewed, or dried states and their juices can be consumed as well. High protein foods are meat, poultry, fish, eggs, all dairy products (except butter), beans, and nuts. Cake that is made with milk and eggs is a high protein food. Pasta and bread contain a great deal of protein, but low protein forms of each can be found. If you are eating a protein-limited diet, you must be careful that you are getting enough calories from the other foods you are eating. Together with swallowing difficulties and other problems, eating can become so troublesome that weight loss and malnutrition can result.

89. Is NutraSweet safe for people with Parkinson disease?

Aspartame (NutraSweet) is composed of two amino acids: aspartic acid and the methyl ester of phenylalanine. When aspartame is absorbed, about 10% of the dose is converted to methanol, which is then converted to formaldehyde, then to carbon dioxide and water. All of these conversions occur by normal metabolic processes. These same processes are used in converting the methanol found in many fruits, fruit juices, vegetables, and wine, to carbon dioxide and water. Thus, methanol is a natural by-product of the metabolism of many commonly eaten foods. In fact, a glass of tomato juice provides about 5 times as much methanol as a similar amount of diet soft drink containing aspartame. The amounts of methanol from many foods, or the lesser amounts from aspartame, are rapidly metabolized, do not accumulate in the body, and do not reach harmful amounts.

The small amounts of methanol formed by the metabolism of aspartame have been alleged, in uncontrolled studies, to be a factor in diseases such as PD. The presence of phenylalanine in aspartame has likewise been alleged to block the absorption of levodopa and to aggravate PD. However, PD existed before aspartame was invented, and there is no evidence that aspartame causes or aggravates PD.

The safety of aspartame has been established, and consumption of diet soft drinks or other foods containing aspartame is not associated with adverse health effects. The level of daily consumption that is judged to be safe by the FDA is 50 milligrams per kilogram (mg/kg) of body weight per day. At this level, for example, a 150 lb (60 kilogram) person would need to consume sixteen 12-ounce cans of a beverage containing aspartame to reach this level of intake.

90. Is caffeine good for people with Parkinson disease?

There are studies that suggest that caffeine protects against PD. The studies indicate that if you drink several cups of coffee a day, and have been doing so for many years, you are 30% less likely to have PD. However, care must be taken in how these data are interpreted. Although it was found that people who drank coffee or other caffeine-containing beverages such as tea, cocoa, and cola, had lower incidences of PD, other explanations are possible. It could be that as PD develops, with its tremors and sleep problems, people with PD begin to avoid caffeine. Another explanation might be that people with a tendency to develop PD have a physiological or psychological intolerance to caffeine.

In one study, men who drank large quantities of coffee or caffeinated beverages had a lower risk of PD than men who drank only a little. The study suggested that it is the caffeine consumed before the onset of PD that provides the protection: caffeine consumed after PD develops provides no protection. In women, the protective effects of caffeine are harder to evaluate. In moderate amounts, caffeine, in women, appears to offer some protection from PD. However, at increased levels of consumption, the benefit is lost, and a reverse effect is observed. This may have a biological explanation, or perhaps women have a different susceptibility to PD. Obviously more studies are needed.

If you enjoy drinking coffee or tea, continue to do so. If you don't, don't start drinking it because it might prevent PD. And, if you have PD, drinking or not drinking coffee will not make a difference. Starbucks is a wonderful place; but it's not the answer to PD.

91. Is smoking good for people with Parkinson disease?

Several studies suggest cigarette smoking may protect against developing PD. Thus, if you smoke one or two packs a day and have been doing so for many years you are about 50% less likely to have PD. These studies indicate the degree of protection is related to the number of packs smoked per day, and the number of years smoked. There is no evidence, however, that once PD begins, smoking is protective. Researchers do not agree on the process by which cigarettes have a protective effect. At different times, it has been proposed that certain chemicals in cigarette smoke, not yet identified, may have a protective effect. Other researchers have noted that nicotine, by stimulating nicotine receptors in the brain, may lessen some of the symptoms of PD. Some point out that cigarette smoking, by decreasing life span, may "kill off" those people who would have developed PD. Other researchers point out that PD is a slowly evolving disease and the disease begins years before it is diagnosed. These researchers think that an early loss of desire to smoke may actually be an early symptom of PD. Instead of viewing smoking as "neuro-protective," they believe that people who do not take up smoking or stop smoking may already have PD.

92. Is hormone replacement therapy (HRT) good for Parkinson disease?

At menopause, women stop making estrogen and hormone replacement therapy (HRT) was developed to alleviate troubling symptoms. For instance, estrogen replacement can relieve hot flashes that, in some people, can be debilitating. This is of concern to women with PD, whose risk for osteoporosis is increased. Also, although studies are not conclusive, there is evidence that estrogen may protect against PD. Evidence for this is small but tantalizing—statistically, more men than women have PD: 55 men for every 45 women. Scientists believe estrogen may modulate dopamine receptors. In fact, some pre-menopausal women report their PD drugs are ineffective during ovulation (the middle of the menstrual cycle) and shortly before the start of their monthly menses, when estrogen levels are low.

Statistically, more men than women have PD: 55 men for every 45 women.

For years, HRT for women has consisted of an estrogen made from the urine of pregnant horses (Premarin) and progestin, a synthetic form of the hormone progesterone (Provera). The combination is called Prempro. The treatment was originally given to relieve such symptoms as hot flashes, but later to reduce bone thinning and heart disease. Estrogen alone relieved symptoms, but produced a small increase in the risk for uterine cancer, so the synthetic progestin was added to lower this risk. But did estrogen or an estrogen-progestin combination really reduce the risk of heart disease? Two studies cast doubt on the safety of both estrogen and estrogen-progestin therapies. However, many doctors do not think the results of these studies are a reason to stop HRT.

At this time, the best advice is to weigh all the possibilities with your doctor. I do not recommend that a woman take estrogen solely because it *may* slow the progression of PD. There are too many variables, too many potential side effects of HRT.

93. Will I need a cane?

Walking difficulty is common in PD, and for many it's a major problem. Walking difficulty results from a combination of slowed movement, incomplete movement (shorter steps) and postural instability. In PD, your steps get shorter, you start to shuffle, your arms no longer swing, and your turns become harder; you hesitate, freeze, and fall. Sometimes you're propelled forward (anteropulsion), sometimes you're propelled backward (retropulsion). In advanced PD, before starting to walk you may hesitate with your feet seemingly glued to the ground. Start hesitation is a form of FOG. Visual tricks and perceptual cues can sometimes help you overcome the "freeze" and resume walking; however, your walking difficulty may eventually increase to the point where you need to consider a cane or a walker.

There are differences between canes and walking sticks. Canes are cut at the level of the low point of your arm swing. If your posture is stooped, a cane that is too low may exaggerate the curve which, in turn, perpetuates your small, short steps. A walking stick, if it's the right height (shoulder level), forces you to walk straight; however, it's harder to learn how to properly use a walking stick than a cane, and your balance may not be as good as with a cane. If your balance is good and you don't fall, then a walking stick may be for you, but if your balance is poor and you fall frequently, a cane might be better for you. Walking sticks can be found in many outdoor sports supply stores and they come in a wide variety of woods. Try using one that you like or maybe different walking sticks for different occasions! Canes, too, come in more than just one variety. Adjust the height so you are comfortable. If you are having difficulty with balance or if you tend to fall, then a three-pronged cane may be optimal. They are harder to use, but give you more support and better traction. Remember, however, falls often occur when you turn. If you are in the habit of picking up your cane before you turn, the cane will not help—it must be touching the ground to support you! Learn to place your cane on the floor and use it for support before you turn. The people who make the "U-Step" walker also make a laser cane. The laser projects a line on the floor and allows you to step over it. This is especially helpful for people who have freezing of gait.

If maintaining your mobility requires more than a cane or walking stick, you need a walker. Some people are horrified by the idea of using a walker because they associate walkers with being an "invalid," but a walker is a device to keep you mobile—and if you're mobile, you're not an invalid, whatever physical challenges you may have. It beats being stuck in a chair or in bed— just ask anyone who can't use a walker which they would prefer. A physical therapist or your doctor can advise on what type of walker will work best for you. Your walker should be light but sturdy—light enough to transport, but sturdy enough so that when you turn, you don't first pick up your walker without thinking. If

Some people are horrified by the idea of using a walker because they associate walkers with being an "invalid," but a walker is a device to keep you mobile— and if you're mobile, you're not an invalid, whatever physical challenges you may have.

you do this, you will fall, with the walker falling on top of you. Walkers with large wheels are easier to turn than walkers with small wheels. Walkers with ball bearings may be even better, especially the "U-Step" walker. Remember to adjust your walker's height; if it is too low and forces you to bend, you will negate the benefits of the walker. To view the laser cane and the U-Step walker go to www.ustep.com.

Finally, wheelchairs come in a variety of types and can be very useful for trips outside the home. Most public museums, parks, movie theatres and concert halls are prepared to handle wheelchairs and usually give folks in wheelchairs preferential treatment. Using a wheelchair will conserve your energy so you can better enjoy the event and the people who are with you. Motorized wheelchairs are an even better way to get around and still maintain your independence. These devices come not only in many styles, but also in different colors. Batteries allow them to travel long distances before recharging, and that can be as easy as just plugging into a wall outlet overnight. They are expensive, but insurance may cover part, if not all, of the cost. Second-hand ones that have been reconditioned may be a good value, too. Be sure to shop around and find one that is the right size and has the necessary features to be useful for you. Think of your wheelchair as mounted infantry. Your wheelchair is the train, the truck, or the helicopter that takes you to where you need to go.

94. When should I apply for disability?

Many employers offer varying types of disability insurance as part of their benefits packages to employees. If you are fortunate enough to be covered by such a policy, the human resources department of your employer will be able to guide you. There are also numerous other insurance policies for long-term disability and, if you have one, the insurance company should direct you as to how to apply. The one benefit that all Americans have paid into is Social Security, which, in addition to retirement assistance, also offers disability benefits. However, the government's definition of disability is very strict: the disability must last longer than 12 months, must be "medically determined," and must prevent the person from doing any class of work, not just the type of work they did before the disability. Two types of assistance are available: Supplemental Security Income and Social Security Disability Insurance. The first, Supplemental Security Income (SSI), assists anyone with low income who meets the government's definition of disability. It has restrictions on income and assets, and the maximum benefit (at this time) is only $545 a month.

The second type of assistance, Social Security Disability Insurance (SSDI), is a type of insurance for which the applicant must qualify. To qualify, the applicant must be under the age of 65, have paid into Social Security for at least 20 of the last 40 calendar quarters, and his or her disability must have begun while he or she was paying into the fund. The amount of benefit the person may receive is calculated based on both earnings and the amount paid into the insurance. At present time, the maximum benefit payable is $1,300 per month. There is also a mandatory five-month waiting period from the time the disability occurred before applying for this benefit. After age 65, the disability benefit will revert to retirement benefit, but the amount paid will remain the same.

Both benefits require an application to be submitted to the Social Security Administration. Once the Social

Security Administration has verified all of the non-medical information, the application is sent on to Disability Determination Services (DDS), which will verify the medical aspects of the disability. It is a good idea to have copies of all medical records documenting your disability and submit them with the application. The DDS will request any additional records they may need and may request an independent medical examination to verify the disability. The evaluation can take up to 145 days, and may even be denied for lack of medical information. If it is denied, the decision must be appealed within 60 days and new medical information given to support it. No benefits are paid during the review or appeals process. If there is any question about the procedure or whether you are entitled to disability, it's best to consult with a disability lawyer.

If there is any question about the procedure or whether you are entitled to disability, it's best to consult with a disability lawyer.

If the claim is accepted, people receiving SSI are usually entitled to receive Medicaid benefits. However, Medicaid is administered by the state, and the payments are so low that many physicians will not accept them. If SSDI is awarded, there is a two-year wait to apply for Medicare. Medicare has two parts: one part covers hospitalization, including all in-patient care, and the second part covers medical doctors and out-patient expenses. The hospitalization part is covered by Social Security and costs the individual nothing. The second part, however, requires a monthly premium. Neither the hospitalization nor the medical expense policies cover the cost of prescription drugs.

95. How can I make my home safer?

In your home, look at the areas where you walk frequently: from your bed to your bathroom, down the hall, to the kitchen, to the front or back door, and to your favorite chair in the living room. Make sure that those areas are safe for walking: remove loose throw rugs, add extra lighting, and put night-lights where they will be the most helpful. Have rails installed along long stretches of hallway. Using motion detection devices on lamps in sitting areas will ensure light to see by and will reduce the hassle of turning them on manually. Move any obstacles out of the way to reduce chances of tripping and falling. Buy a long-handled mechanical tool for picking up things that drop to prevent unnecessary bending. A cordless phone that can be carried in a pocket or in the basket of a walker is a boon for catching calls without running to the phone. A television remote control with large buttons is another "user-friendly" device.

If you have stairways in your home, make sure that the carpet isn't loose and that the steps aren't cracked. Putting reflective tape along the edges makes the steps more visible, especially at night. Make sure that the handrails are firmly attached and sturdy. Adding a second handrail on the other side may also prove useful. If doorknobs become troublesome, change them for lever-type door handles. Keys can be more easily managed if they are kept in a plastic holder that provides a grip as well as storage. Be sure to have good lighting at entryways—motion detectors or timers are useful here, too.

Most accidents in the house occur in the bathroom. Slipping and falling are the most prevalent here, and thus, prevention is the goal. Small throw rugs on the floor can slip and slide or bunch up and cause falls. They should be removed and replaced with larger rugs that have non-slip backings. Adding grab bars to tub and shower walls helps to prevent falls, and grab bars near the toilet will help with getting up and down. An elevated toilet seat may also help with moving your bowels, as well as making it easier for you to get on and off the seat. Be sure to put a rubber bath mat in the tub or shower to prevent slipping on the wet surface.

Adding a bath stool or chair with rubber suction tips makes bathing easier, too. Buy soap on a rope or use shower gel from a tube to prevent slippery bars of soap from getting away. If faucet handles in the sink or shower are difficult to grasp, replace them with larger lever types. Hand-held shower heads on long hoses are convenient and easy to use and can help you ensure that the water temperature is correct before you get in.

Make sure that there are no glass containers in the bathroom: shampoo, hand cream, and mouthwash should all be purchased in plastic tubes or bottles. Exchange glass tumblers for paper cups to minimize the chances of breaking. Toothbrushes with fat handles make oral hygiene easier to manage, and electric shavers reduce the risk of nicks and cuts. A night light is essential in the bathroom and a large bell on the countertop or toilet tank makes it easy to summon help.

Bedrooms should be comfortable, private areas that invite rest and relaxation. Be sure to have clear access to the bed, free of shoes or other clutter, and that the path to the bathroom is open. Because PD makes turning in bed slow and difficult, a blanket support at the foot of the bed allows feet to move freely. Satin sheets allow you to turn more easily. A firm mattress also provides you with the support and leverage you need to turn more easily. If you're still having difficulty turning in bed, it is probably because you do not raise your arm high enough to flip yourself over. Ask your partner to watch you turn in bed. If you're not raising your arm high enough you're not going to turn easily.

Slippers should be easy to slip onto your feet but not off, and they should have non-slip soles. A box of tissues, an accessible flashlight, and an unbreakable container of water on the nightstand will also come in handy. A night light with a motion detector that can switch on with the least movement can be useful.

For men, a urinal can reduce trips to the bathroom. If a commode is necessary, be sure that it is placed as close to the bed as possible, with toilet tissue within easy reach. A plastic cloth on the floor beneath the commode can prevent spoiling the carpet in case of accidents or spills. A chair for dressing is indispensable, and it should have arms for ease in getting in and out. Other dressing aids include a long-handled shoehorn, a buttonhook, and a zipper-pull.

As for the kitchen, there are gadgets that help open jars of many different sizes, from catsup bottles to large mason jars. Electric can-openers are a boon, but you should find one that is easy to use and hard to break. Electric knives may also seem like a good idea, but they're not: if you slip, the cut is likely to be bigger and bloodier. Cutting boards that have suction feet can prevent slipping while cutting, and knives with larger handles are easier to use. If handles are not big enough for you to grip comfortably, they can be built up by taping on several layers of foam rubber until they fit your hand. Plastic handles that fit over half-gallon containers of juice or milk make the cartons easier to use.

Cooking food in a crock pot allows different combinations of meat and vegetables to be cooked at the same time, producing tender, flavorful meals with a minimum of effort and reducing the possibility of burning either the food or the cook! Microwave ovens have

Cooking food in a crock pot allows different combinations of meat and vegetables to be cooked at the same time, producing tender, flavorful meals with a minimum of effort and reducing the possibility of burning either the food or the cook!

simplified cooking for everyone, but be sure that the oven is easily accessible to minimize spilling hot liquids or foods. An electric broom makes cleaning up the floor a breeze, and the new soft cloth sweeping systems are better than a broom and dustpan.

Meal times for people with PD can be frustrating. Take the time you need to eat, don't hurry: hurrying can result in choking! Chew your food thoroughly before trying to swallow. If you're having trouble chewing, lift up your chin! People with PD have a tendency to bend their neck (without realizing it) and this results in your chin touching your chest. If you try chewing with your chin touching your chest you'll notice it's harder than chewing with your chin up. You're using the same muscles, but keeping your chin up gives them a mechanical advantage. If you can't remember to chew with your chin up, try keeping your elbows on the table. This is not what your mother taught you, but keeping your elbows on the table automatically forces your chin up. For some people, eating smaller meals more frequently is helpful.

If soup is on the menu, use a large handled mug and drink it. Spoons may be more effective than forks for picking up food from your plate, and if your spoon has a large handle, it will be easier to use. Ask to have your meat cut into bite-size pieces in the kitchen so you don't have to struggle to cut it at the table. Drinking straws work well when tremor makes drinking difficult. Never fill a cup or glass more than three quarters full: it's less likely to spill. A large bore straw rather than a narrow one is better. A damp washcloth makes a great napkin, especially when finger foods are served. A dining chair with arms makes it easier for the person with PD to steady their elbows and arms while eating.

A strategically placed towel can protect your clothes from an accidental spill.

Shopping for clothes to wear can be a problem. Navigating through crowded malls, trying on clothes in small fitting rooms, and waiting in line to pay for your purchases takes the fun out of shopping and leaves a person with PD frustrated and exhausted. Instead, turn to mail-order catalogs and shop for clothing at home. Several companies carry items of clothing that are designed to be easier to put on and take off and still look very attractive. Men can wear pull on shirts, like the 3-button knit sport shirts, or in cold weather they can wear turtlenecks: turtlenecks look great and are easy to wear.

If dress shirts are necessary, try short sleeve shirts, few people notice the absence of buttons or cuff-links. Clip-on ties can substitute for regular ties, which require you to tie a knot, and many clip-ons are indistinguishable from regular ties. For sportier or casual clothes, there are good looking, pull-on pants with elastic waists that eliminate bothering with buttons or zippers. Shoes that close with Velcro are easier to wear than shoes that close with laces. And Velcro, unlike laces, does not break. Slip-on loafers are an equally good choice. Some people need shoes with rubber soles to grip the floor. Some people, especially people who freeze, need leather soles, soles that don't stick on carpets or catch on uneven surfaces and cause you to fall. Whether you need rubber or leather soles will be determined by trial and error. You must try both and see which is best. Women can wear skirts and slacks with elastic waists. They can also wear knit shirts, loose blouses, or pull-on sweaters. Bras that fasten in the front are simpler to put on. Bathrobes should be ankle length at most: floor length robes cause falls. Shoes should have flat or low heels and be easy to put on or take off.

96. How can I meet other people with Parkinson disease?

Remember that you are not alone! The PD community has a large and extensive support network. There are national organizations that sponsor support groups throughout the country for PD patients and their families. Many hospitals and regional health centers also have support groups, and many patients have started groups of their own. A support group can be an important asset to your survival—a lot can happen when a group of determined people rally around one uniting cause! In addition to sharing their experiences with you, members of support groups can often teach you about services available in the community and other local resources. People in support groups usually stay well-informed on the newest and best types of treatments, or may know when and where a new trial or study on PD is taking place. Support groups work to educate the community or promote public policy that benefits people with PD. Support groups may not be for everybody, but there are many different kinds, including some for young-onset PD and some for caregivers, so there might be one that is useful for you.

If a support group is not for you, there are numerous internet-based PD groups that can be accessed at your convenience. Given the nature of the Internet, however, caution is always wise. A wealth of information is available online, but you should always carefully consider the source and accuracy of the information. If it sounds too good to be true, it probably is.

97. Can I safely take a vacation?

If you (or you and your partner) decide to take a vacation, to "get away from it all" for awhile, you must first decide what type of vacation you want. Do you want to travel far? Go to a resort? Take a cruise? Enjoy nature? See an exotic part of the world? These are all possibilities. It may take a bit of extra planning, but you may be pleasantly surprised at the options that are available. Airlines make special efforts to accommodate people with disabilities; you just need to let them know ahead of time what kind of accommodation you need. If your destination is a particular resort or resort area, inquire whether the hotels have special facilities or can make accommodations to fit your requirements. Many cruise lines design cruises for people with disabilities and have medical staff on board to deal with any problems that might arise. Some travel agents specialize in arranging trips and vacations for people with special requirements. A helpful travel agent can find group tours planned especially for people with physical problems or pave the way for independent travel by helping you to connect with the services that you need to succeed. A travel agent can also find the right transportation, shuttles, and services to get you safely to the airport and assist you to get around in unfamiliar airports or make smooth transitions from one means of travel to another; a good agent will find the way to ensure safe arrival at your hotel or arrange appropriate transportation for sight-seeing at your destination. The agent can even arrange to rent special equipment when you reach your destination or make the arrangements to transport equipment with you. If you want to get away and see the world, don't let PD stop you!

98. How long can I remain independent?

No one should have to give up living in his or her own home until it becomes an absolute necessity for safety or health reasons. If your mother has PD, and she is living alone, you must sit down and talk with her about the situation and what she needs to do to stay in her own home. There may be modifications that can be made to make it easier for her. For instance, if the house has an upstairs, then arrangements might be made for her to live downstairs, or if she must go upstairs, then a stair-lift might be installed. Making a shower more accessible so she doesn't have to step into a tub for bathing can also make a difference. Most communities do offer services for the elderly or people with disabilities. They range from special transportation to shopping or doctor's appointments to home health care or visiting homemakers. Services available in your mother's community can probably be found in the phone book—some phone books have separate sections that list providers and their phone numbers and addresses. If your mother goes to a PD support group, they will be able to tell her what is available and who to call. Check with local chapters of national PD organizations to see what information they maintain on services in your area. Sometimes a county social worker can evaluate your mother's needs and make recommendations for services. Often, municipal and county services are stretched beyond their own limits and there may be waiting lists for their services. You could make your own arrangements to have someone come to help clean the house or maintain the yard or possibly have a friend of your mother come to visit her on a regular basis.

Eventually, though, you or your parent may no longer be able to live independently. No one wants to go to a convalescent or nursing home, and no one wants to send his or her partner or parent to one, really. But there comes a time when it is impossible to lift and turn a PD patient, impossible to bathe or clean up after him or her, and impossible to get a good night's sleep to prepare to do it all over again for another day, and even more impossible to care for him or her if the patient has developed dementia. Everyone has heard the "horror stories" about nursing home care, but living at home without proper care is a horror story, too. In a convalescent home, there are strong people to help bathe the patient, hot food and help to feed the patient, people to get the patient up out of bed and clean up behind him/her, even social activities for entertainment—and the care is given 24 hours a day, 7 days a week. So the decision to place a parent or partner in a nursing home must be seen as providing better care for the patient, an opportunity to make the patient's life a bit more comfortable.

Convalescent or nursing homes need to be chosen as carefully as choosing a neighborhood to live in or a school to attend. Locating the right one can be a challenge. As soon as you know that placing someone in a nursing home will be necessary, you need to begin planning. Your doctor or the hospital may be able to give you a list of homes, or you might turn to a national agency for long term care and ask for their recommendations. Churches and fraternal organizations may also offer care. Visit several, interview the director, talk to the nurses, and observe the patients. Find out how many registered nurses are on staff, how many licensed practical nurses, how many nurses' aides are employed, and whether they are permanent employees or are provided by a temporary agency. If the staff is from a temporary agency, they may not be as committed to the home as regular staff employees. Ask whether there is a social worker on staff and try to meet that person. Ask about the doctor on staff and

Find out how many registered nurses are on staff, how many licensed practical nurses, how many nurses' aides are employed, and whether they are permanent employees or are provided by a temporary agency.

find out if he/she will work with the patient's doctor, especially on the PD issues. Ask your own doctor about his/her recommendations for nursing homes and whether he knows the doctors at a particular home you're considering. Make a list of questions you feel are important regarding the care of your parent or partner and compare the answers from several nursing homes. Find out what services are covered and if there are any additional charges for some services that you may need to pay for. Consider carefully the financial implications for the patient and the family. Know as much as you possibly can before making a decision on which nursing home or care facility you choose.

99. How can I protect my assets?

Planning ahead for future care and establishing healthcare directives is a thoughtful consideration for your family. Having someone to talk about it with is important. When it comes to medical care, a living will can not only make your wishes known, but will guarantee that they will be followed. If you feel you may be unable to make decisions about future health care, you can create a durable power of attorney for health care (also known as a health care proxy) and designate a person you trust to make those decisions for you. A form for a living will can be obtained from a lawyer, a hospital, a stationery store or even off the Internet. Be sure it is properly filled out. You must sign the document in the presence of witnesses (which, depending on state laws, might need to be different people from the person named in the document), and some states also require that the signatures be notarized.

If taking care of financial matters is a concern, a durable power of attorney for finances can be useful. Again, check the requirements of your state for filing and registering these instruments. The power of attorney will allow you to appoint someone to handle paying your bills and managing your accounts while you are ill. It can give as broad or specific duties as you specify. However, the power granted in a durable power of attorney for finances ends at your death; the person you appoint will not be able to make arrangements for your funeral expenses. To do this requires a will. A will can be basic, no frills, or complex; it does not necessarily need to be prepared by a lawyer, but it may be helpful to have the advice of a lawyer if your estate or wishes are more complex. It does require you to appoint an executor, whose job it is to make sure your instructions are carried out; it must be dated and signed by you in front of several witnesses who are not named in the will. Much more information on this topic is easily available, either on the Internet, in libraries, or from your attorney.

100. When will there be a cure?

At the beginning of the 20th century, average life expectancy for an American was 46 years: 50% of people died before they were 46 years old, too young to develop PD. In 1900, children died of diphtheria, meningitis, polio, whooping cough, and tetanus. Fifty years later, children were immunized and vaccinated. These diseases, seemingly as incurable as PD, disappeared.

Although the cause or causes of PD are unknown, much is known about how specific substances injure cells in the brain, including the dopamine cells. And, since the introduction of levodopa and the dopamine agonists, much has been learned about how the brain works. Drugs such as levodopa, the dopamine agonists Mirapex and Requip, and the MAO-B inhibitors rasagiline and selegiline, alleviate and improve PD.

As more is learned about the brain, these approaches will be improved. Thus, it has been learned that the early use of the dopamine agonists reduces and delays the appearance of symptoms such as wearing off or "peak dose dyskinesias." Newer, longer-acting agonists may have an even more dramatic effect. PD cannot yet be cured, but its rate of progression may be slowed and some of these drugs may slow the progression of PD.

As surely as we conquered tuberculosis, syphilis and polio, we'll conquer PD.

In 1900, people with tuberculosis, syphilis, or polio, asked the same questions as people with PD today ask: When will there be a cure? The answer was then as now—I don't know, but I'm confident it'll come. As surely as we conquered tuberculosis, syphilis and polio, we'll conquer PD. Parkinson seems more difficult to conquer because, unlike the other diseases, we don't know the cause, but our technology is more advanced than in 1900, our doctors better trained, and our resources greater: I believe a cure will come—and in our lifetime.

Organizations

Muhammad Ali Parkinson Center
  240 West Thomas Road
  Website: www.maprc.com
  Website: www.thebarrow.org
  Phone: 602-406-4309
  Fax: 602-406-6131

Parkinson Action Network
  300 North Lee Street, Suite 500
  Alexandria, VA 22314
  E-mail: info@parkinsonaction.org
  Phone: 1-703-518-8877 (1-800-850-4726)
  (CA: 1-707-544-1994)
  Fax: 1-703-518-0673

Parkinson Alliance
  211 College Road East, 3rd Floor
  Princeton, NJ 08540
  E-mail: admin@parkinsonalliance.net
  www.parkinsonalliance.net
  Phone: 1-609-688-0870 (1-800-579-8440)
  Fax: 1-609-688-0875

Parkinson Disease Foundation
  710 West 168th Street
  New York, NY 10032-9982
  E-mail: info@pdf.org
  www.parkinsons-foundation.org
  Phone: 1-212-923-4700 (1-800-457-6676)
  Fax: 1-212-923-4778

Parkinson Institute
675 Almanor Avenue
Sunnyvale, CA 94085-2935
E-mail: outreach@parkinsonsinstitute.org
www.parkinsonsinstitute.org
Phone: 1-408-734-2800 (1-800-786-2958)
Fax: 1-408-734-8522

Parkinson Research Foundation
P.O. Box 20256
Sarasota, FL 34276
Website: www.parkinsonresearchfoundation.org
Phone: 703-821-1975
Fax: 866-317-0593

National Parkinson Foundation
1501 N.W. 9th Avenue
Bob Hope Research Center
Miami, FL 33136-1494
E-mail: mailbox@parkinson.org
www.parkinson.org
Phone: 1-305-547-6666 (1-800-327-4545)
(FL: 1-800-433-7022)
Fax: 1-305-243-4403

Michael J. Fox Foundation for Parkinson Research
Grand Central Station
P.O. Box 4777
New York, NY 10163
www.michaeljfox.org
Phone: 1-212-213-3525

American Parkinson Disease Association
1250 Hyland Boulevard, Suite 4B
Staten Island, NY 10305-1946
E-mail: apda@apdaparkinson.org
www.apdaparkinson.org
Phone: 1-718-981-8001 (1-800-223-2732)
(CA: 1-800-908-2732)
Fax: 1-718-981-4399

Worldwide Education & Awareness for Movement Disorders
204 West 84th Street
New York, NY 10024
E-mail: wemove@wemove.org
www.wemove.org
Phone: 1-212-875-8312 (1-800-437-MOV2 (6682))
Fax: 1-212-875-8389

Brain and Organ Donation

NINDS sponsored:
Dr. Wallace Tourtellote, Director
National Neurological Research Specimen Bank
VMAC (W127-A)-West Los Angeles
11301 Wilshire Boulevard
Los Angeles, CA 90073
(310) 268-3536

Francine M. Benes, M.D., Ph.D., Director
Harvard Brain Tissue Resource Center
McLean Hospital
115 Mill Street
Belmont, MA 02478
(617) 855-2400
www.brainbank.mclean.org.8080

Privately sponsored:
National Disease Research Interchange (NDR)
1880 JFK Boulevard, 6th Floor
Philadelphia, PA 19103
(800) 222-NDRI (800 222-6374)
(215) 557-7361

University of Miami Brain Endowment Bank
Department of Neurology (D4–5)
1501 N. W. Ninth Avenue
Miami, FL 33101
(800) UM-BRAIN (800 862-7246)
(305) 243-6219

**Publications and Information from National Institute
of Neurological Disorders and Stroke (NINDS):**

Parkinson Disease: Hope Through Research
An informational booklet on Parkinson disease compiled by the
NINDS.

La Enfermedad de Parkinson: Esperanza en la Investigacion
A Spanish-language public information booklet on Parkinson
disease/Informacion de la Enfermedad de Parkinson.

Parkinson Disease Research Agenda
NINDS Parkinson Disease Research Agenda, March 2000.

Parkinson Disease Backgrounder
A backgrounder on Parkinson disease.

September 1999 Parkinson Testimony
NINDS Director's September 1999 Congressional testimony on
National Institutes of Health Parkinson disease research.

Parkinson Disease: A Research Planning Workshop
Summary of a 1995 Parkinson disease research-planning workshop
sponsored by the National Institutes of Health.

Researchers Find Genetic Links for Late-Onset Parkinson Disease
December 2001 news summary on recent findings in Parkinson
disease genetics.

Parkinsonian Symptoms Decrease in Rats Given Stem Cell Transplants
January 2002 news summary on embryonic stem cells used in a
mouse model for Parkinson disease.

Workshop Summary: Cognitive and Emotional Aspects of Parkinson Disease
Summary of workshop, "Cognitive and Emotional Aspects of
Parkinson Disease: Working Group Meeting," held January
25-26, 2001.

Third Annual Udall Centers of Excellence for Parkinson Disease Research Meeting
Summary of Third Annual Udall Centers for Parkinson Disease
Research meeting. NINDS, the National Institute of Neurological
Disorders and Stroke, is the leading supporter of biomedical research on the
brain and nervous system.

Parkinson Disease Research Web
A National Institutes of Health disease-specific web site to facilitate research
on Parkinson Disease. NINDS is the leading supporter of biomedical
research on the brain and nervous system.

2002 Parkinson Disease Testimony
NINDS opening statement to the Senate Committee on Appropriations,
Subcommittee on Labor, Health and Human
Services, Education, May 22, 2002.

Helpful Phone Numbers:

American Healthcare Association: 1-202-842-4444

Americans with Disabilities Act Regional and Technical Assistance Centers: 1-800-949-4232

The National Council On the Aging, Inc.: 1-202-479-1200

Elder care Information and Referral Services: 1-800-677-1116

National Council on Disability: 1-202-374-1234

American Red Cross: 1-800-435-7669

American Occupational Therapy Association: 1-301-652-2682

American Physical Therapy Association: 1-800-999-2782

American Massage Therapy Association: 1-847-864–0123

Health-Related Web Sites:

www.acurian.com (enrolling clinical trials, news and information on drugs in development, and Federal Drug Administration-approved treatments)

www.parkinsonscare.com (National Parkinson Foundation's caregiver Web site)

www.ahca.com (American Healthcare Association)

www.achoo.com (Achoo Health Director)

www.HealthAtoZ.com (search engine for health and medicine)

www.medhelp.org (MedHelp International)

www.caregiving.org (National Alliance for Caregiving)

www.globalrx.com (FDA-approved mail-order service)

www.geohealthweb.com (Geo Health Web)

www.caregiver911.com (Caregiver Survival Resources)

Helpful Videos:

The Educated Caregiver

A three-part videotape series dealing with care giving, a nice complement to *The Comfort of Home: An Illustrated Step-By-Step Guide for Caregivers.* To order, contact Life View Resources, Inc., P.O. Box 290787, Nashville, TX 37229-0787, or phone 1-800-395-5433.

The Parkinson Education Team

From the Young-Onset & Care Partner Support, Group Denver, CO. To order, contact Karl Ferguson at 1-303-830-1839 or e-mail parrockies@aol.com. Cost $20. Run time 1 hour and 25 minutes.

8 Weeks to Optimal Health
Videotape companion to the book of same title by Andrew Weil, M.D. A holistic approach to better nutrition and improving the mind/body connection. At video stores or from www.amazon.com.

Tai Chi for Seniors
A 30-minute video introduction to the Chinese exercise form. Order by phone at 1-909-943-2021.

The Meaning of Health: Healing and the Mind
A PBS video production narrated by Bill Moyers. Order online from www.amazon.com.

Gentle Fitness
An award-winning videotape of six short routines to improve flexibility, balance, and breathing. Order from 732 Lake Shore Drive, Rhinelander, WI 54501, or order by phone at 1-800-566-7780 (www.gentlefitness.com).

Sit and Be Fit
Videotape companion to the PBS exercise series. Special edition for PD. Phone orders: 1-509-448-9438 or Fax: 1-509-448-5078 (www.sitandbefit.com).

Catalogs featuring products to make living with Parkinson disease easier:
Sammons Preston: 1-800-323-5547
Sears-Home Health Service: 1-800-326-1750
J.C. Penney Easy Dressing Fashions: 1-800-222-6161
Adaptability: 1-800-243-9232
Caring Concepts: 1-800-500-0260

Glossary

Ablative procedures: procedures that remove damaged tissues through ablation, or destruction using heat sources.

Acetylcholine: a chemical that acts to transmit nerve impulses in the brain, the peripheral nerves, the heart, the gut, the bladder, and the muscles.

Activities of daily living (ADLs): activities usually performed for oneself in the course of a normal day including bathing, dressing, grooming, eating, walking, using the telephone, taking medications, and other personal care activities.

Agent Orange: an herbicide developed for the military and thought by some to cause PD.

Akathisia: an inner sense of restlessness, like an "ants in the pants" feeling.

Akinetic-rigid syndromes: movement disorders marked by stiffness and a lack of movement.

Alogia: unwillingness to speak.

Alpha-synuclein: protein contained in Lewy bodies and targeted by PD (also called Parkin 1).

Alzheimer's disease: a brain disorder characterized by memory loss and dementia. It is not related to Parkinson disease, but has some similar symptoms.

Amantadine: a drug originally developed for flu symptoms. It has been found to increase dopamine production and suppress acetylcholine in Parkinson patients.

Amygdala: the "rage center" of the brain.

Amyloid plaques: protein deposits around blood vessels.

Anemia: low red blood cell counts that result in fatigue and dizziness.

Anergia: lack of physical and mental energy.

Anhedonia: lack of pleasure in daily activities.

Anosmia: loss of smell.

ANS: see Autonomic nervous system

Anteropulsion: a feeling of being pushed forward.

Anticholinergics: drugs that block the activity of acetylcholine.

Antihistamine: a medicine used to treat allergies and hypersensitive reactions and colds; works by counteracting the effects of histamine on a receptor site.

Antioxidants: substances that bind free radicals and prevent them from damaging cells.

Anxiety: a condition of fearfulness and stress that can exacerbate PD-related symptoms.

Apomorphine: dopamine agonist that is rapidly broken down, or metabolized, in the liver.

Apoptosis: cell death.

Arteriosclerosis: the narrowing of medium and small-sized arteries by cholesterol and by changes in the artery's muscular wall.

Aspiration: choking; accidentally inhaling food.

Asterixis: sudden relaxation of a group of muscles which causes the limb to suddenly jerk.

Ataxia: difficulty with walking and balancing.

Atherosclerosis: the narrowing of a large artery by cholesterol.

ATP: the chemical fuel that powers most of the cell's activity.

Atrophy: a weakening of the muscles that extend or straighten your spine.

Atypical poliomyelitis: one of the diagnoses for the mysterious "sleeping sickness" pandemic of the early 1900s (see von Economo's Encephalitis).

Autonomic nervous system (ANS): the portion of the brain and nervous system that governs or regulates the body's internal environment.

Babinski response: name given to test response when the patient's big toes curl up after the doctor scratches the soles of the feet with a pin.

Ballismus: a movement disorder that consists of sudden flinging of an arm or a leg.

Basal ganglia: a series of interconnected regions of the brain including the striatum, globus pallidus, and thalamus.

Benign essential tremor: a common movement disorder related to anxiety. It is sometimes confused with PD because the principal symptom is shaky hands.

Biological marker: a specific protein or genetic change that distinguishes a particular disease or condition.

Botox (botulinum toxin): a large protein molecule that blocks the release of acetylcholine onto muscles and can stop the secretion of acetylcholine by the salivary glands.

Bradykinesia: a primary symptom of PD that consists of slow movement, an incompleteness of movement, a difficulty in initiating movement, and an arrest of ongoing movement are associated with this slowness. Bradykinesia is the most prominent and usually the most disabling symptom of PD.

Bromocriptine: a dopamine agonist.

Calmodulin: a protein found in neurons of the substantia nigra that are targeted by PD.

Carbidopa: a drug that is given with levodopa to reduce its side effects.

Cardinal symptoms: the four main symptoms of PD.

Cataracts: a condition in which the lens of the eye becomes cloudy and obscured, usually relieved with surgery.

Cerebellum: the coordinating center of the brain that acts as a "first responder" to information from the nervous system.

Cerebral cortex: the conscious, thinking brain.

Ceruloplasmin: a protein which carries copper in the body.

Chelators: drugs which detoxify and remove metal ions from the brain.

Cholinergic receptors: enzymes in cells that attach to acetylcholine.

Chorea: movement disorders characterized by dance-like, flowing movements of arms or legs, often involving every part of the body. Also called dyskinesia.

Chromosomes: collections of genes that compose DNA. All people have 23 pairs of chromosomes in every cell.

Clinical trials: carefully monitored scientific studies of new drugs or treatments using human subjects.

Coenzyme: substances that are chemically related to other substances that have a specific effect. Coenzymes often are examined to determine if they can create similar effects to known enzymes without side effects.

Cogwheel rigidity: PD symptom in which an arm or a leg "catches" during movement, resembling the way a cog catches in a wheel.

Constipation: difficulty in passing stool.

Contralateral: on the opposite side.

Corpus striatum: an area of the brain named because of the large number of fibers that cross it—giving it a stripped or braided appearance (the name comes from the Latin "stripped-substance").

Cortex: the thinking part of the brain.

Corticobasilar degeneration: a movement disorder with rigidity symptoms similar to those of PD.

CSF: a watery fluid, continuously produced and absorbed, which flows in the ventricles (cavities) within the brain and around the surface of the brain and spinal cord.

Deep brain stimulation: a treatment in which a probe or electrode is implanted and used to stimulate a clearly defined, abnormally discharging brain region to block the abnormal activity.

Deep tendon reflex tests: one of the functions of medical evaluation, conducted by tapping with a rubber reflex hammer on the tendons at your jaw, elbows, knees, and ankles.

Delusion: a belief in something with no basis in reality.

Dementia: a loss of previously acquired thinking skills.

Dementia pugilistica: a condition caused by repeated blows to the brain that some boxers develop over several years.

Depression: chronic feelings of sadness, despair, and helplessness.

Detrusor: the bladder is a smooth muscle, called the detrusor.

Diabetes: a condition in which the body cannot process sugar, either because it lacks insulin or because the body has become resistant to insulin.

Diphenydramine: Antihistamine (trade name Benadryl) used to treat allergic reactions involving the nasal passages (hay fever) and also to treat motion sickness.

Diuretics: medications that help to rid the body of excess water.

DNA: DNA, or deoxyribonucleic acid, is the hereditary material in humans and almost all other organisms.

Dopa decarboxylase: the enzyme that changes levodopa to dopamine.

Dopa responsive dystonia (DRD): an inherited disorder that starts in the teens, 20s and 30s first described in Japan by Professor Segawa, often called Segawa's disease.

Dopamine: a chemical messenger in the brain; loss of dopamine is a key factor in PD.

Dopamine agonist: drug that exerts its pharmacologic effects by directly activating dopamine agonist receptors.

Dorsal vagal nucleus: the "head" or "chief" nucleus of the para-sympathetic nervous system (calming center).

Drooling: the discharge of saliva from the mouth.

Drowsiness: a state of impaired awareness associated with a desire or inclination to sleep.

Dynamic balance: the ability to right yourself when stumbling or pushed.

Dysarthria: difficulty forming or pronouncing words.

Dyskinesia: dance-like involuntary movements. Dyskinesia may involve the face, the tongue, the head and neck, the trunk, the arms and legs.

Dysphagia: difficulty with swallowing.

Dystonia: involuntary muscle spasms resulting in awkward and sustained postures, which may be painful. Dystonia can involve the eyes, neck, the trunk, and the limbs.

Edema: swelling of the legs.

Electromyogram (EMG): an electrical recording of the muscle firing.

Encephalitis lethargica: the sleeping sickness that occurred early in the 20th century with some symptoms resembling PD.

Enteric nervous system: the nervous system that regulates the bowels.

Epidemic delirium: one of the diagnoses for the mysterious "sleeping sickness" pandemic of the early 1900s (see von Economo's Encephalitis).

Epidemic schizophrenia: one of the diagnoses for the mysterious "sleeping sickness" pandemic of the early 1900s (see von Economo's Encephalitis).

Essential tremor: a disease sometimes confused with PD.

Extremity: the endpoints of the limbs, e.g. the toes, feet, fingers, and hands.

Facial mask: a symptom of PD in which the muscles of the face can no longer move, creating an expressionless, mask-like demeanor.

Fava: Fava is Italian for bean and refers specifically to the broad bean. Fava beans are the main commercial source of the drug L-DOPA.

Free radicals: toxic molecules that arise from the breakdown and oxidation of foods and naturally occurring body chemicals.

Freezing: a PD symptom in which the person is unable to complete a normal motion, such as moving a leg while walking.

Gene therapy: therapy that seeks to replace or repair a defective gene that causes a disease or condition.

Genes: long strands of four molecules that determine the way in which proteins are made. Genes are the basis of heredity.

Gengenhalten: involuntary resistance to passive movement of the extremities.

Ginseng: a herb that has been used to stimulate the adrenal gland and thereby increase energy. It also may have some beneficial effect on reducing blood sugar in patients with diabetes mellitus.

Glaucoma: a disease of the eyes in which fluid accumulates behind the eye and presses on the optic nerves, in time leading to blindness.

Glial derived neurotrophic factor (GDNF): a specific growth or trophic factor, the lack of which cause neurons to die.

Globus pallidus: a portion of the basal ganglia affected in PD. This region of the brain is known to be overactive in animal models of PD.

Green tea: tea made from leaves that are not fermented before being dried.

Half-life: a measure of the duration of the drug's action.

Hallucinations: a delusion in which a person sees or hears things or people that don't exist.

Hemiballismus: violent involuntary movements resembling someone repeatedly throwing a shot-put, or hurling a discus following destruction of the STN is by a stroke or tumor.

Hereditary: passed down through the genes from parents to children.

Hippocampus: the portion of the brain that stores memories.

Huntington disease: an inherited disorder of the brain.

Hydrocephalus: disorder in which there is too much cerebrospinal fluid in the ventricles of the brain.

Hyperkinetic: excessive movement.

Hypertension: high blood pressure.

Hypomimia: a mask-like expressionless face caused by rigidity of facial muscles.

Hypophonia: softness of voice stemming from rigidity in the muscles of the larynx and lungs.

Hypothalamus: a region in the brain that controls all the glands and the autonomic nervous system.

Hypotonic bladder: an underactive bladder where in which the bladder fails to empty completely and the urine dribbles out the urethra.

Impotence: inability to maintain an erection sufficient to complete sexual intercourse.

Incontinence: inability to hold one's urine or bowels.

Infarct: death of a region of the brain supplied by a blocked artery.

Intention tremors: Tremors appearing or exaggerated as you reach for a specific object.

Intercostal muscles: muscles between your ribs, your respiratory muscles.

Kinetic tremor: tremor that is present when you move your hands

L-dopa: see Levodopa.

Lacunes: small infarctions which individually cause no symptoms, but cumulatively may cause a variety of symptoms that mimic PD.

Lee Silverman Voice Therapy: a method of training a person to strengthen his or her voice by singing loudly or shouting.

Lesion: a breakage or damaged area in tissue.

Levodopa: a drug used to treat PD that is transformed into dopamine by the substantia nigra.

Lewy bodies: small, iridescent pinkish spheres found in the dying nerve cells of people with PD.

Libido: desire for sex.

Locus ceruleus: part of the brainstem involved in and which may account in part for the sleep disturbances involved in PD.

Magnetic resonance imaging (MRI): a technique that creates 3-dimensional images of body structures using strong magnetic fields.

Manganese fumes: fumes generated in the process of welding that some believe may cause PD.

Merocrine glands: sweat glands that discharge their secretion, sweat, directly on your skin's surface.

Micrographia: a PD symptom in which the affected individual's handwriting becomes small and illegible due to decreasing control over hand muscles.

Mitochondria: cellular energy sources.

Monoamine oxidase B (MAO-B): an enzyme in the mitochondria which increases with age, resulting in an increased production of toxic free radicals.

Motor exam: physical examination that checks a person's ability to move and respond to stimuli.

Movement disorder: any of a number of conditions that affect a person's ability to move normally, or that cause abnormal, involuntary movements.

MPTP: a narcotic-like drug known to cause permanent PD symptoms.

MRI: see Magnetic resonance imaging.

MSA with ataxia: a combination of MSA and atrophy of the cerebellum.

Multiple-system atrophy: a set of movement disorders with PD-like symptoms.

Muscarinic receptors: cholinergic receptors in the bladder.

Myleopathy: a gait disorder that results from pressure on the upper or cervical spinal cord.

Myoclonus: a movement disorder that consists of quick, jerking movements that can involve one finger or the entire body.

Neupro: is used to treat early signs and symptoms of Parkinson's disease.

Neurofibrillary tangles: twisted fibers of a tau protein inside the neurons in dying brain cells.

Neuroleptics: the first drugs successfully used to treat the symptoms of psychosis and schizophrenia (also called major tranquillizers).

Neurologist: a physician specializing in diseases of the brain and nervous system.

Neuropathy: damage to the nerves in feet.

Normal Pressure Hydrocephalus: is a rise in cerebrospinal fluid (CSF) in the brain that affects brain function.

Nurturin: a specific growth or trophic factor, the lack of which cause neurons to die.

Olfactory cortex: located within the medial temporal lobes the olfactory complex allows us to identify odors.

On time: in PD, the times in which a person is able to move normally without displaying symptoms of the disease.

On-off: in PD, the condition of alternating "on" (asymptomatic) periods with "off" periods in which symptoms such as freezing or dyskinesia are evident.

Ophthalmologist: a physician specializing in eye disorders.

Ophthalmoscope: a lighted tool for examining the eye.

Optic nerves: nerves that transmit sight.

Opticokinetic nystagmus (OKN): response to a test of your eyes' ability to follow figures or lines on a tape that is past them in which your eyes beat rapidly, the absence of which suggests the presence of PSP.

Orbicularis oris: the lips.

Orthostatic hypotension: a condition in which the body's blood pressure regulating mechanism fails to respond adequately to abrupt changes, e.g., when a person experiences dizziness upon standing up.

Overflow incontinence: continual leakage of urine due to the bladder being constantly full.

Pallidotomy: a surgical procedure that can decrease dyskinesia, reduce tremor, and improve bradykinesia by interrupting the flow of neurochemicals from the globus pallidus.

Panic: a heightened state of anxiety combined with physical changes in the autonomic nervous system.

Panic attack: a sudden onset of panic with no apparent cause.

Paralysis agitans: an agitated or trembling paralysis.

Paranoia: a belief that people are seeking to harm you.

Parkinsonism: a class of movement disorders with similar symptoms. Parkinson disease is one of these disorders.

Pergolide: a dopamine agonist.

Pesticides: chemicals toxic to insects that prey upon crops. Some pesticides are also harmful to humans.

PET scan: see Positron emission tomography.

Physiologic tremor: is the tremor that is present in everyone, brought out with stress, a fever, or with an overactive thyroid gland.

Pigmented melanin granules: a naturally occurring antioxidant found in the substantia nigra that give the nigra, the "black substance," its name.

"Pill-rolling" tremor: PD symptom that looks like rolling a cigar, coin, or pill between thumb and index finger.

Platelets: blood cells that cause clotting of blood and wound healing.

Pleura: the double-walled sac enclosing the lungs.

Positron emission tomography (PET): a scanning technique that allows the creation of 3-dimensional images of body structures, particularly the brain.

Postural hypotension: a drop in blood pressure upon sitting or standing.

Postural instability: a lack of balance or unsteadiness while standing or changing positions.

Postural reflexes: reflexes that allow one to maintain balance.

Pramipexole: a dopamine agonist.

Presbyopia: a condition of the eye in which the length of the lens changes with age.

Progressive disorder: a condition that has progressively more severe symptoms over time.

Progressive supranuclear palsy: a movement disorder with symptoms similar to PD.

Psychosis: a mental disorder in which delusions and hallucinations are combined; the person is convinced that unreal things or people truly exist.

Putamen: the target of the neurons in your substantia nigra.

Pyridoxine: vitamin B-6.

Rasagiline (Azilect): is an irreversible inhibitor of monoamine oxidase used as a monotherapy in early Parkinson's disease.

Resting tremor: a trembling of the hands or feet that occurs only when not in motion.

Restless legs syndrome: an uncomfortable, aching sensation that is relieved if you constantly move your legs; usually occurs during sleep or while resting.

Retropulsion: the need to take steps backward in order to begin moving forward.

Rigidity: *Stiffness* or tightness of the muscles.

Romberg test: a test that observes whether a person asked to stand still sways backward or forward.

Ropinerole: a dopamine agonist.

Schizophrenia: a mental illness often characterized by auditory hallucinations.

Sebaceous glands: glands in the skin and scalp that secrete oil.

Seborrheic dermatitis: a scaling condition of the skin that occurs in PD patients.

Selective norepinephrine reuptake inhibitors (SNRIs): antidepressant drugs which increase brain levels of norepinephrine, not serotonin.

Selective serotonin reuptake inhibitors (SSRIs): the most commonly prescribed antidepressant drugs; they help both anxiety and depression.

Senile gait: shrinkage or atrophy of the brain with a loss of the neurons that regulate walking.

Sepsis: blood poisoning.

Serotonin: a brain chemical that is related to anxiety and depression.

Shaking Palsy: paralysis agitans or trembling paralysis.

Shy-Drager: Multi-system atrophy with ANS involvement.

Sialorrhea: drooling.

Sleep apnea: a breathing disorder characterized by brief interruptions of respirations during sleep.

Start hesitation: or "failure of gait initiation" is a PD symptom characterized by the inability to start walking.

Static balance: balance in which the body maintains equilibrium for one position.

Statins: supplements used to lower cholesterol that may also slow the progression of PD.

Stem cell: a primitive cell that has the ability to divide countless times and to give rise to specialized cells.

Striatonigral degeneration (SND): the most difficult of the MSAs to distinguish from PD; characterized by early appearance of a flexed neck and a poor response to levodopa.

Striatum: a portion of the brain, connected with the substantia nigra, which is affected by PD.

Strider: the shrill, high-pitched sound that occurs when vocal cords close completely.

Substantia nigra: a portion of the brain with darkly pigmented cells that is a principal location affected by PD.

Subthalamic nucleus: an area of the brain located below the thalamus that acts as a "brake" on the substantia nigra.

Supra nuclear: a neurologic disorder of unknown origin that gradually destroys cells in many areas of the brain, leading to serious and permanent problems.

Sustention or Postural tremor: tremor present when the limbs or trunk are kept in certain positions and when they are moved actively.

Sweat glands: tubular glands that are found nearly everywhere in the skin of humans and that secrete perspiration externally through pores to help regulate body temperature.

Tardive (meaning delayed) dyskinesia: movements in drug-induced PD that appear after the drug is started, or sometimes after the drug is stopped.

Tetrachlorodibenzodioxin (TCDD): prototype for a class of halogenated aromatic hydrocarbons, which appear to have a common mechanism of action and to produce similar effects, although they differ in potency; achieved notoriety in the 1970s when it was discovered to be a contaminant in the herbicide Agent Orange and was shown to produce birth defects in rodents.

Thalamotomy: a surgical procedure targeting the thalamus designed to stop tremors.

Thalamus: portion of the brain that receives impulses from the nerves and transmits it to the conscious brain.

Tics: involuntary muscle twitches or movements.

Tonic foot: the sole of the foot gripping the ground (also known as "grasp").

Tremor: involuntary trembling, usually of the hands or head.

Tricyclic antidepressants: are medicines that relieve mental depression.

Urinary retention: inability to urinate even when the bladder is full.

Urodynamics: a series of tests that assess how well a patient can control his or her bladder.

Urologist: a physician who treats problems of the bladder and urinary tract.

Vascular Parkinson: condition caused by a cumulative effect of multiple "silent" or "minor" strokes affecting the striatum, globus pallidus, thalamus, cerebellum, and midbrain that cause symptoms similar to PD.

Vestibular nucleus: a region of the brain stem that receives messages from the inner ears and eyes regarding balance.

von Economo's encephalitis: see Encephalitis lethargica.

Wearing off: a condition in which medications for PD slowly become less effective over time.

Welding: the process of joining metals together using a filler and an electric arc.

Wilson disease: an inherited disorder in which a mutation in a gene on chromosome 13 leads to a deficiency in a protein called ceruloplasmin.

Young Onset Parkinson Disease (YOPD): PD that begins at or below 40 years of age.

Index

Index

Index